SPORTS INJURIES

SPORTS INJURIES

A practical manual for trainers, coaches, players and schools

by

David S. Muckle M.B., B.S., F.R.C.S.

ORIEL PRESS

First Printed in Great Britain 1971

ISBN 0 85362 096 2
Library of Congress Catalogue Card Number 79-122524

The illustrations were specially drawn by
D. P. Hammersley and E. Patterson

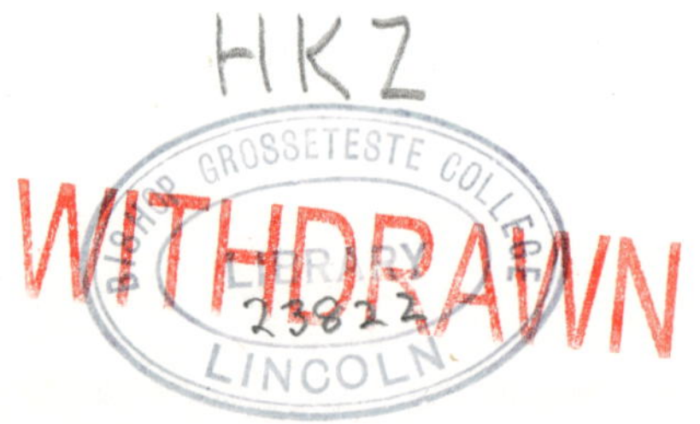

Published by Oriel Press Limited
32 Ridley Place
Newcastle upon Tyne
England NE1 8LH
Printed by Knight & Forster, Leeds

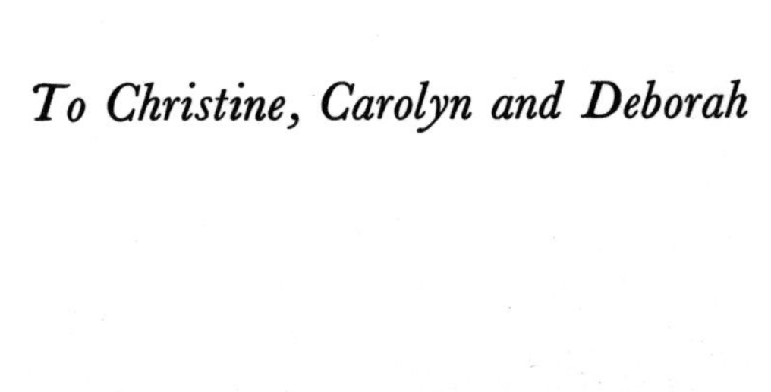

To Christine, Carolyn and Deborah

FOREWORDS

This book deals comprehensively with most of the injuries that are liable to occur in sport. It is extremely well illustrated and the clinical expositions and treatment of the lesions are clearly explained to those who undertake immediate care. The descriptions lie within the easy grasp of the people under whose jurisdiction such lesions are liable to happen. Explanations are full and carefully documented from a regional point of view, and the index facilitates easy search for information. It should prove of use in many of the F.A. coaching courses and is a first rate reference book for football trainers whether amateur or professional and could very well grace the shelves of the physiotherapists associated with all sports. Its lucidity should appeal to all.

FENTON BRAITHWAITE, O.B.E., F.R.C.S.
Consultant Surgeon,
Royal Victoria Infirmary, Newcastle upon Tyne,
Director, Newcastle United A.F.C.

This book will serve as an excellent guide to everyone connected with sports injuries. As an ex-professional player I realise the importance of prompt diagnosis and treatment of any injury, however minor, to promote a rapid return to full activity. This book will be a great boon to the many minor clubs and associations that lack full medical facilities and I am sure will appeal to sportsmen of all kinds.

JOE HARVEY,
Manager—Newcastle United A.F.C.
Ex-Captain Newcastle United.

ACKNOWLEDGEMENTS

I would like to thank D. P. Hammersley for the excellent medical drawings, completed in the Dept. of Photography, Newcastle University, and E. Patterson for the sports action drawings. I am indebted to Margaret Stevenson, MA who typed and checked the manuscript, Eileen Richardson of Oriel Press for her patience in arranging the layout of this book, Mr. C. K. Warrick FRCS and staff of the Dept. of Radiology, Royal Victoria Infirmary, Newcastle, and Mr. J. K. Stanger FRCS, Orthopaedic Dept., Royal Victoria Infirmary for permission to reproduce the X-rays, Mr. J. R. G. Edwards FRCS, Plastic Unit, Royal Victoria Infirmary for his advice, Mr. Stanley J. Knott for his helpful criticism and advice, and finally the staff and players of Whitley Bay F.C. with whom I have been associated both in playing and in a medical capacity over the last five years.

CONTENTS

1 Care of the Injured 1

2 Sports Injuries 14

3 The Structure of the Body
(*Anatomy and Histology*) 99

4 Functions of the Body
(*Physiology*) 125

5 General Data 134

1. CARE OF THE INJURED

Emergency Treatment of the seriously injured

URGENT . . . maintain AIRWAY by removing false teeth, elevating the tip of the jaw or grasping the tongue in a dressing to prevent obstruction by the TONGUE FALLING BACKWARDS onto the laryngeal inlet. Keep the face to the side and downwards to allow mucus, blood and vomit to escape out of the mouth. Foreign bodies may have to be pulled from the throat with the finger.

URGENT . . . CONTROL HAEMORRHAGE by the application of a pressure dressing OVER THE BLEEDING AREA. THIS IS THE SAFEST AND BEST METHOD. OBSERVE PULSE, ONSET OF PALLOR, anxiety and sweating (indications of SHOCK). A tourniquet is rarely necessary unless bleeding is profuse from a large wound. The use of a tourniquet is often exceedingly DANGEROUS, since if it is applied too LOOSELY haemorrhage is INCREASED, and if it is applied too TIGHTLY serious **damage** can be done to the VESSELS AND NERVES. Remove the tourniquet as quickly as possible; up to half an hour (or more) can only be excused by very exceptional circumstances. REMEMBER PRESSURE FROM THE FINGERS AND THUMB, or a PRESSURE DRESSING, is the main line of treatment.

URGENT . . . Treat every case of injury as a FRACTURE until it is proved to be otherwise. PROTECT AND IMMOBILISE ALL injured players until the diagnosis is made. SPLINT THEM WHERE THEY LIE, do NOT waggle the limb around, this produces further damage and bleeding. ALWAYS USE GENTLENESS AND CARE IN HANDLING ANY BROKEN LIMB.

Have a STRETCHER handy for transportation.

If a fracture is obvious do not examine the parts, WATCH THE CIRCULATION by colour and pulse below the fracture.

Fractures of the lower limb and forearm are treated by external splinting, the damaged area being surrounded by soft padding. For fractures of the arm and elbow a well-applied sling is recommended. When a FRACTURED SPINE IS SUSPECTED the LESS the patient is handled, the better. Transport on a FIRM SURFACE, e.g. a wooden board or door. If such a board is not available it is occasionally justifiable to roll the patient gently on to a blanket for transportation. With an INJURED CERVICAL SPINE (NECK) the face should point UPWARDS, with the HEAD SUPPORTED BY SANDBAGS OR ROLLED BLANKETS. These patients must NEVER be turned to the side or face down. Patients with FRACTURED THORACIC OR LUMBAR SPINES should be transported in the SUPINE (face up) position if possible. Transport with care and gentleness, DISTURB THE PATIENT AS LITTLE AS POSSIBLE. NEVER, NEVER, GIVE A DRINK OR FOOD TO AN INJURED PERSON—it DELAYS ANAESTHETIC and may be INHALED and CAUSE DEATH.

KEEP CALM, DO NOT FUSS THE INJURED. THE LESS HELPERS THE BETTER (within reason).

Emergency Care of the Unconscious

1. Rapidly assess the level of consciousness, if patient responds when questioned or pinched he/she is semiconscious.
2. Ensure adequate airway by placing on side with mouth down. Remove teeth, blood clots and other foreign bodies.
3. Observe respiration rate, pulse, colour of face and limbs.
4. If breathing stops apply MOUTH TO MOUTH RESPIRATION AT ONCE.
5. Observe pupils. Unequal in size or rapidly dilating indicates brain compression from swelling or blood. EMERGENCY. TRANSPORT TO HOSPITAL AS QUICKLY AS POSSIBLE.
6. If breathing is not noisy carry player on stretcher.
7. If noisy due to air bubbling through blood or mucus, place face down with mouth over the end of the stretcher. Now elevate the foot of the stretcher to drain fluid out of mouth and lungs.
8. Observe for lack of movement. This may indicate paralysis.
9. Slowing pulse and laboured breathing are serious signs.
10. Observe pulse, respiration and size of pupil every few minutes.
11. NEVER GIVE FLUIDS. If fluid enters the LARYNX AND LUNGS it will cause death.
12. DO NOT FORGET SPINAL and OTHER INJURIES MAY ALSO EXIST, transport with care.
13. Even after a few seconds of unconsciousness the player should NOT be allowed to continue, take to hospital or doctor for examination.
14. After a minor head injury trainer or captain should question the player concerned regarding current score or location of event and other simple questions. His reply may indicate confusion or disorientation. (If so, treat as 13).

Mouth to Mouth Respiration
External Cardiac Massage

1. Feel for a **pulse** at the wrist or neck. With death bleeding suddenly ceases from the wound.

2. IF NONE FELT AND THE PERSON STOPS BREATHING COMMENCE . . .

3. MOUTH TO MOUTH RESPIRATION. Clear mouth and throat of debris, lie person on back and extend the neck by tipping the head backwards, (this opens up the airway), pinch the subject's nose (to stop air coming down), TAKE A DEEP BREATH AND BLOW INTO THE SUBJECT'S MOUTH UNTIL THE CHEST RISES. Take mouth away and air will rush out of the patient. REPEAT EVERY SIX SECONDS, i.e. ten times approx. per minute. (A handkerchief with a hole can be placed over the patient's mouth or a plastic airway used). If no response after a few seconds an observer, preferably with medical experience, should commence . . . .

4. EXTERNAL CARDIAC MASSAGE. Kneel beside the patient with elbows extended and place both hands (crossed) over the lower part of the sternum (central breastbone) and press firmly but gently backwards depressing the chest wall for 1″ (2–3 cm.), then release. A pulse should be felt at the wrist, neck or groin. REPEAT AT THE RATE OF approx. 60 per minute. AFTER EVERY THIRD OR FOURTH BEAT ALLOW THE PERSON DOING MOUTH TO MOUTH RESPIRATION TO INFLATE THE LUNGS (approx. 12 per minute).

5. CONTINUE WITH ALTERNATE RESPIRATION AND MASSAGE UNTIL MEDICAL HELP IS AVAILABLE.

6. Do not press too hard against the chest wall in massage because rib fractures and cardiac bruising may occur. BE FIRM AND GENTLE, HOWEVER.

7. Observe the pupils, if they start to constrict then a good

outcome is to be expected.

N.B. The patient should be on a hard surface whenever possible, if not, place a wooden board beneath the patient. Depression of the sternum of ½″ (1—1.5 cm.) only in children, when one hand can be placed behind the chest to facilitate compression.

External cardiac massage is tiring and persons should alternate between mouth to mouth respiration and massage every FIVE minutes.

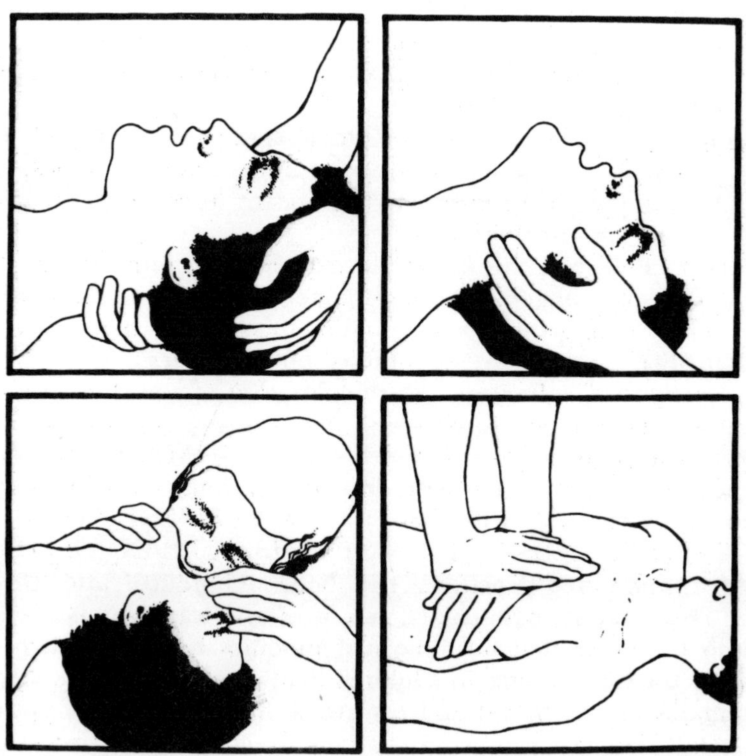

Diagnosis of a Fracture

This section must be read before dealing with individual fractures.

PAIN . . . variable, usually sharp and severe, especially in large bones, swelling and bruising always accompany a fracture but are not diagnostic.

DEFORMITY . . . usually characteristic of a fracture, but not invariable.

ABNORMAL MOBILITY . . . if found is diagnostic of a fracture.

BONE TENDERNESS . . if tenderness is accurately localised to the surface of the bone and not the soft tissues above, then bone tenderness is sure sign of a fracture even if all other signs are lacking.

LOSS OF FUNCTION . . . unlike sprains or bruises of soft parts, fractures involving the extremities render it impossible for the patient to exert any significant force by pushing or pulling against resistance.

CREPITUS . . . this is the grating sensation imparted to the examining fingers when the bone ends move against each other. It is better not to produce this sign for bleeding and further damage may be inflicted on the tissues.

Late signs of a fracture are discoloration of the skin (ecchymosis) and fracture blisters.

Fractures may be SIMPLE (closed), or COMPOUND when the bone communicates with the open air, and is thus exposed to contamination with bacteria. COVER THE WOUND OR BONE ENDS WITH A STERILE (CLEAN) CLOTH. In comminuted fractures the bone is broken into three or more parts; in impacted fractures one fragment is driven into the other and no abnormal mobility is present. Greenstick fractures occur in children and one side of the bone remains intact. Spiral and transverse fractures are descriptive of the damage produced. Fatigue fractures (or stress) are produced with excessive use of the limb. In COMPLICATED fractures a nerve, vessel or organ is damaged. THESE ARE SERIOUS fractures and MUST ALWAYS BE CONSIDERED while examining the patient. SHOCK accompanies this type of fracture. Pathological fractures are found in diseased bones.

Confirmation of the fracture is by X-RAY.

TREATMENT. Initially by splintage (as described), then reduction and fixation. Reduction may not be necessary if displacement has not occurred. Minor fractures in non-weight-bearing bones can be treated by crepe or adhesive strapping, but most fractures need immobilisation in plaster of paris. (P.O.P.) Occasionally internal fixation with metallic screws or plates is carried out.

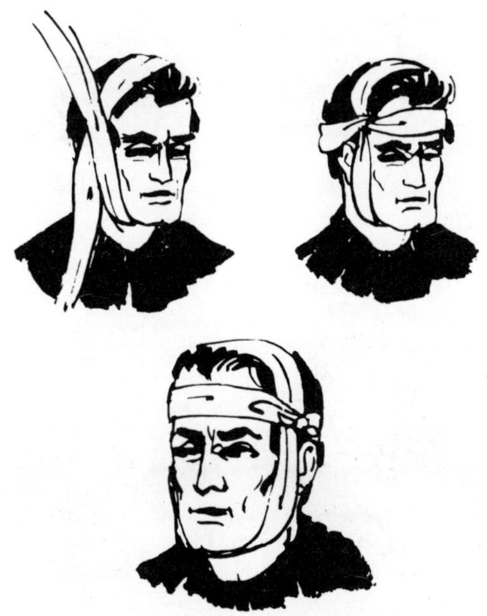

Support for jaw and facial fractures

Diagnosis of Dislocation.

Pain of severe or sickening character near a joint, plus fixity of the joint, deformity, and swelling. In many cases it is difficult to distinguish between a dislocation and a fracture, and both may occur at the same time. Secure the bones involved and transport to hospital for X-ray.

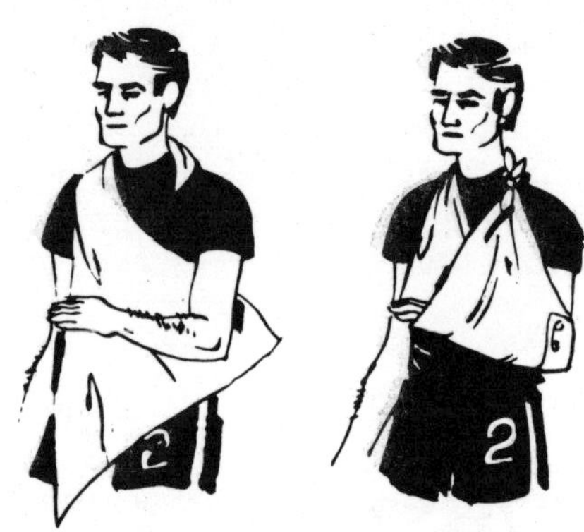

Sling—for elbow and forearm injuries

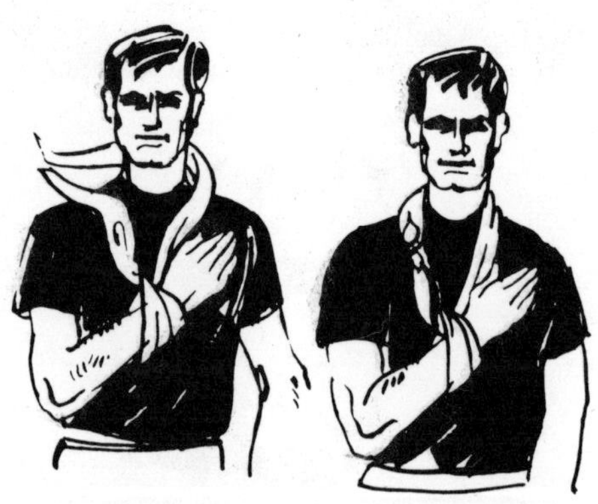

Collar and cuff for shoulder and arm injuries

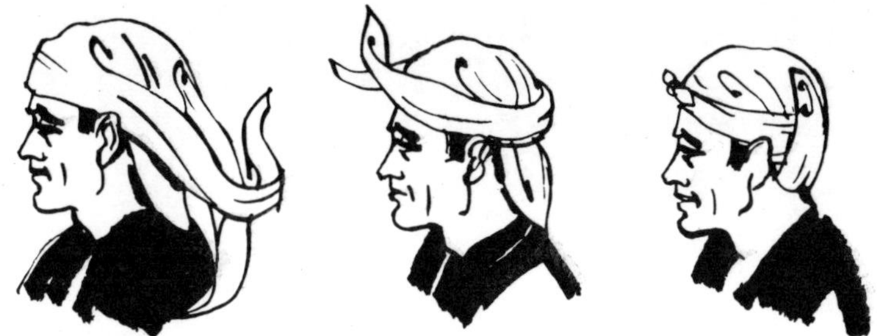

Compression and protective bandage for scalp and head injuries

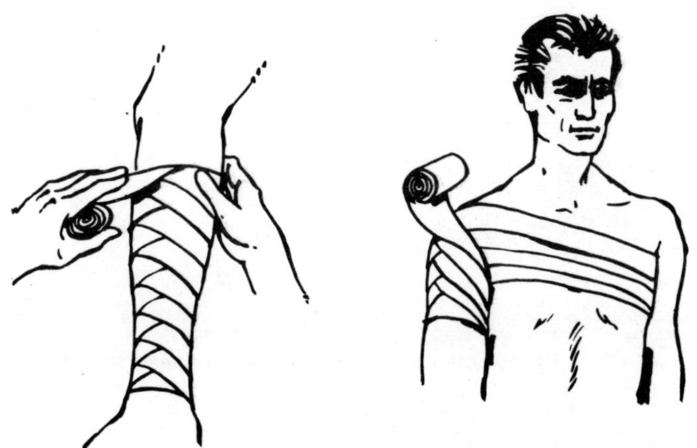

Methods of applying bandages to support or protect parts

METHODS OF APPLYING BANDAGES TO ARM

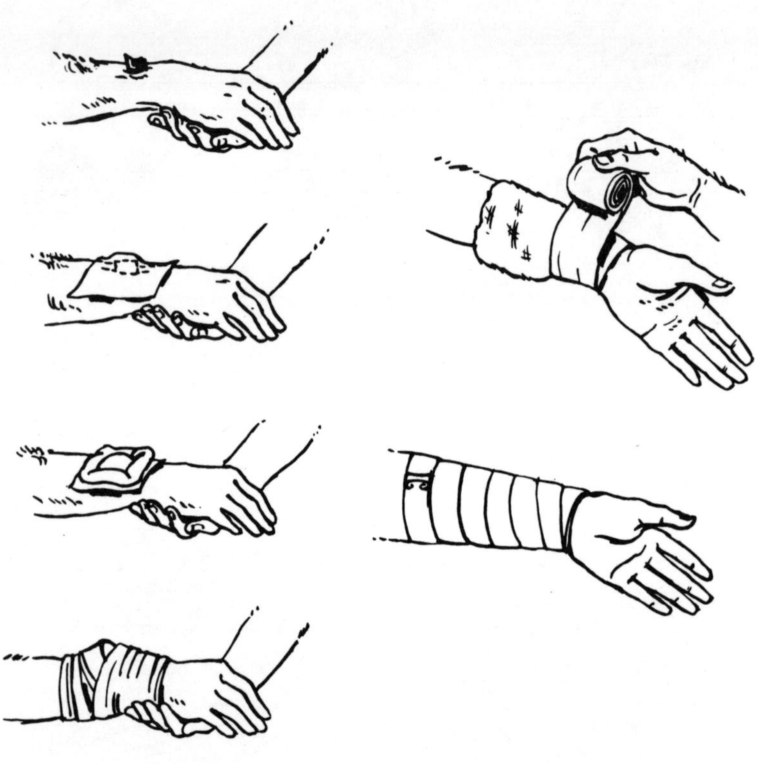

(N.B. Foreign body left in position until hospitalisation)

Damage to an Artery, Diagnosis

Arteries may be damaged directly in a laceration, or by sharp fragments of bones in a fracture. Bruising of the vessel wall is often followed by thrombosis and emboli. In many cases the vessel goes into spasm which reduces or obstructs the circulation, e.g. supracondylar fractures of the elbow. A traumatic aneurysm may develop from a pulsating haematoma, or an arteriovenous fistula result from penetrating trauma (here the blood is diverted to the vein because of the lower pressure in this vessel).

Indications of damage to an artery:

1. Reduced warmth and absence of pulses in a limb below the level of injury are definite indications of arterial damage.
2. Pallor, mottling, blueness (cyanosis), and a waxy appearance of the skin of the hand or foot are indicative of circulatory insufficiency in the limbs.
3. Poor nerve conduction as indicated by weakness or numbness and tingling may indicate arterial damage.
4. A wound near a large vessel should arouse suspicion of vascular damage.
5. Recurrent bleeding from a wound may be a warning that a vessel is injured, it may be a prelude to massive bleeding.
6. Progressive increase in the circumference of a limb provides evidence of a concealed haematoma (blood-clot) and haemorrhage.
7. Signs of shock usually indicate bleeding from somewhere, may be intrabdominal or within the chest.
8. Blood may escape into the urine, bowel, bronchi or other passageways or cavities of the body before becoming obvious.

The treatment is by PRESSURE DRESSING, if possible.

Complete severence of a vessel may lead to less blood loss than a partial severence.

NERVE DAMAGE

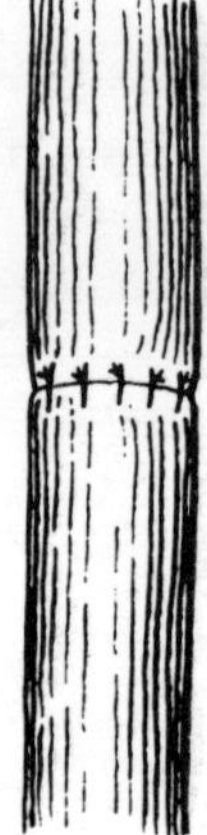

suture of fine outer coat of *nerve* allows nerve fibres (axons) to grow down into severed portion. There may be mixing of sensory and motor fibres at the cut so that poor nerve function results.

ARTERY DAMAGE

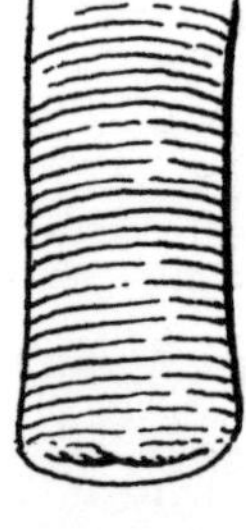

spasm and platelet thrombi (clot) occlude the severed vessel

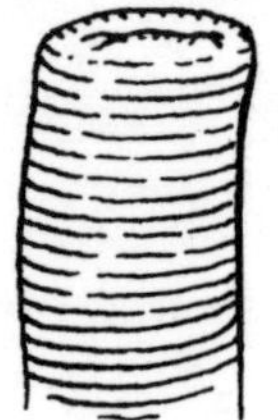

blood loss 30 ml.

Complete

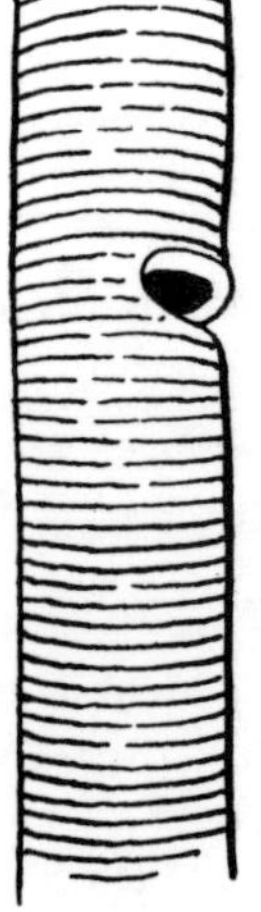

spasm cannot take place, and thrombus formation is poor

blood loss 300 ml.

Incomplete

Experiment to show degree of blood loss with complete and incomplete arterial damage.

Diagnosis of Nerve Damage

The early diagnosis of nerve injuries is vital for successful treatment, although operative repair may be delayed for three or more weeks. Nerve lesions may be produced by stretching, partial and complete rupture. The following signs and symptoms indicate loss of conduction in the major nerves. It should be emphasized that loss of conduction does *not* always indicate complete division of a nerve, bruising and stretching can cause identical findings.

a). The ULNAR nerve. Injury is demonstrated by an inability to feel pain on deep pressure or pin prick over the tip of the little finger. With higher lesions there is inability to flex (bend) the tip of the same finger.

b). MEDIAN nerve. In injury above the elbow pain is not felt with deep pressure or pin prick in the tip of the index finger which also cannot be flexed. The thumb cannot be opposed and a letter 'O' cannot be formed by the thumb and index finger.

c). RADIAL nerve injury is demonstrated by an inability to extend the wrist—there is wrist drop; or difficulty in extending the tip of the thumb.

d). Damage to the EXTERNAL POPLITEAL nerve is indicated by an inability to dorsi-flex the ankle or extend the toes, i.e. there is foot drop.

e). Damage to the POSTERIOR TIBIAL NERVE is indicated by an inability to feel pain over the outer aspect of the foot and an inability to plantar flex the ankle or toes.

f). Damage to the SCIATIC nerve has findings consistent with loss of both d and e.

g). Damage to the main plexus of the arm (BRACHIAL) or lower limb (LUMBOSACRAL) is complex with multiple areas of anaesthesia and weakness in the limbs involved.

2. SPORTS INJURIES

Injury to the Skin

a). ABRASION . . . when only the epidermis and superficial layers of the dermis are damaged. Usually caused by studs, rough ground etc.
Treatment: gentle cleansing with mild antiseptics (Dettol, Hibitane, T.C.P. in water), exposure to air — dressings stick to the oozed serum and are best avoided. Spray with polybactrin (or other antibiotic spray) if necessary. Vaseline impregnated dressings (Tulle gras) should be used if dressings needed (e.g. on the buttock).
Small particles of dirt will cause a tattoo mark in the tissues and need abrasive treatment with a nail-scrubbing brush under local anaesthetic.
b). SIMPLE OR LINEAR LACERATIONS . . . involve dermis, 'clean cut'. Small blood vessels are injured, leading to slight blood loss and formation of haematoma (blood clot) in the tissues.
Treatment: short lacerations, less than $1\frac{1}{2}$–2″, and facial lacerations, are best treated with 'dumb-bell' or 'butterfly' sticking sutures, except where movement is excessive e.g. over joints or at angle of mouth. Longer lacerations need suture with black silk (Casualty Department).
Large haematomas need release by incision or aspiration; spreading agents like hyaluronidase may aid dispersal. Scar tissue will be kept to a minimum if natural skin creases and blemishes are accurately approximated.
c). CONTUSED LACERATIONS . . . have jagged edges, require excision to simple laceration, then suture (as above).
d). PUNCTURE WOUNDS . . . liable to infection, need antibiotics, Tetanus Toxoid, etc.
e). COMPOUND LACERATIONS . . . These may involve an ARTERY, VEIN, NERVE, JOINT, BONE or other important structures. ALL LACERATIONS ARE POTENTIALLY

dangerous and should be gently examined to ascertain damage to other structures as well as the skin. DO NOT POKE INTO A WOUND. If bleeding is excessive apply pressure with pressure dressing (cotton pad and bandage) and elevate the limb (unless fractured). Inquire regarding loss of sensation or movement. Severed tendons, ligaments, or muscles may be obvious. Clear, 'oily' fluid may be escaping from a joint. Deep puncture wounds can penetrate such structures. If in doubt seek medical advice.

Dangers of Skin Injury

Infection is the greatest danger. Usually the bacteria can be controlled with routine antibiotics. ALL ATHLETES, especially in CONTACT SPORTS, should be immunised against TETANUS. Infection with the tetanus organism, found in the soil is commonly fatal. Three small injections confer resistance. Gas gangrene is very occasionally found after sports injuries. Rapid swelling and discoloration of the limb with profound illness are the presenting symptoms.

Injuries to Ligaments

a). SPRAIN . . . is a stretching of a ligament due to the joint being forced into an excessive or abnormal position. Diagnosis—mild pain, tenderness, swelling (slight), restricted mobility in a joint.

Treatment: rest–24 hrs., crepe or stockinette support. If more severe, or recurrent, may need elevation, compression dressing, strapping (adhesive) or P.O.P.

b). PARTIAL RUPTURE . . . occurs when the deforming force continues beyond the strain stage. Diagnosis—as above but symptoms worse.

Treatment: ice, compression, elevation, localisation by ultrasound and possible hydrocortisone (steroid injection). May need strapping or P.O.P.

c). COMPLETE RUPTURE . . . total loss of NORMAL

movement in joint, may be excessive, or limited due to muscle spasm.
Treatment: usually needs suturing in hospital, with P.O.P. for several weeks.
Mild sprains should heal in 1–2 weeks, partial rupture in 3–4 weeks, complete may take up to 6–10 weeks. Recovery sufficient to allow normal training cannot be said to have taken place until there is full range of active joint movements, full passive, no contracture of muscles around the joint, and normal movement patterns. There should be no pain, no tenderness and no laxity at the joint.

Injuries to Tendons

Tendons are enormously strong e.g. the Achilles can support a load of half a ton per square inch. They contain special nerve endings that reflexly inhibit over-contraction of the muscle, but tears do occasionally occur.
a). SPRAIN . . . as in the case of ligament injuries due to a deforming force in abnormal posture or excessive normal position. Diagnosis—as ligaments, but degree of swelling varies with the presence or absence of a tendon sheath. If present, swelling extends along sheath and is more obvious.
Treatment: as above (ligamentous sprain).
b). PARTIAL RUPTURE . . . may be due to a 'pulling' injury or a laceration. There is marked loss of function and no high activity possible.
Treatment: rest and support for 2–6 weeks (may need P.O.P.). STEROID INJECTIONS SHOULD NEVER BE GIVEN as they convert a partial into a complete rupture by interfering with the blood supply and weakening the collagen structure. Often recurrent, partial ruptures can ruin a sporting career.
c). COMPLETE RUPTURE . . . complete loss of power and a palpable gap, common in Achilles tendon, long head of biceps of arm, plantaris, shoulder cuff muscles, long extensor of

thumb and extensors of fingers. Surgical suture necessary, with P.O.P. immobilisation for 4–8 weeks.

d). PERITENDINITIS . . . due to chronic inflammation around the tendon insertion due to overuse (e.g. golfer's or tennis elbow) or adhesions from old injury (usually repeated partial ruptures) as in the peritendinitis of Achilles tendon. Diagnosis—dull aching pain worse after exercise, usually little swelling, tenderness over the tendon concerned.

Treatment: rest, alteration in technique (e.g. less straight-arm backhand strokes in tennis), steroid injection, ultrasound, heat and general physiotherapy.

e). SIMPLE TENOSYNOVITIS . . . produced by unaccustomed activity. Diagnosis—pain and swelling with a characteristic soft crepitus (likened to the creaking of new leather) is palpable to the examining finger, on examination of the tendon.

Treatment: rest and bandage support.

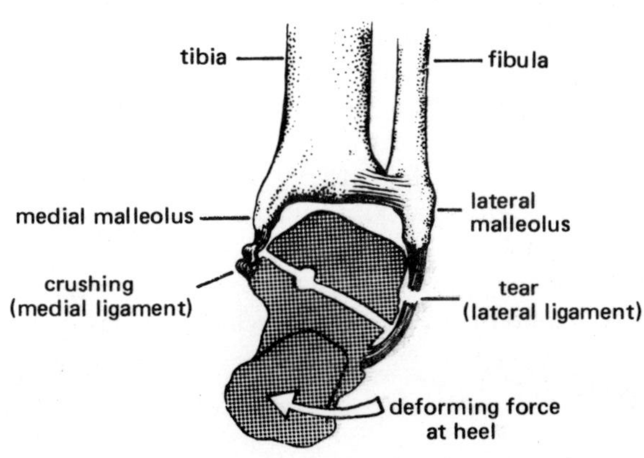

Illustration showing how one injuring force can damage ligaments on both sides of a joint (in this case a severe twisted ankle).

Damage to Muscle

During exercise there is up to a 15-fold increase in blood supply to the muscle, thus any tearing of a vessel is accompanied by marked haemorrhage in the damaged area. Injuries are caused by DIRECT blows ('charley-horse' injury of America), INDIRECT ('pull', 'tear' or 'strain') or OVERUSE (chronic indirect injuries). Damage may be:

a). INTERMUSCULAR: pain, and swelling followed by loss of power and movement. Tends to subside after 48–72 hours. Bruising appears at site remote from the original injury, having tracked down the Intermuscular fascial septa.

Treatment: ice, compression, elevation (I.C.E.) during the acute period. Ice for $\frac{1}{2}$–2 hours while swelling is increasing due to oedema and bleeding. The cold produces a reflex vasoconstriction of the blood vessels supplying the muscle. Always apply ice in a towel etc. and not directly on to the skin. A compression bandage, rest and elevation are maintained for 48–72 hours.

After the acute phase static and passive exercises can be carried out. As power increases (4–21 days depending on injury site) and full extensibility begins to return then active exercises can be undertaken. Heat (short wave diathermy, infra-red etc.) should never be given until the acute phase subsides as swelling will be aggravated, but when used later it relieves spasm and eases pain. Massage may be commenced to promote absorption but should be gentle or myositis ossificans can be produced, it must NEVER be given directly over the injury, and is really only of benefit in chronic lesions as deep frictional massage.

b). INTRAMUSCULAR . . . in which the bleeding takes place within (not between) the muscles. (treatment as a).)

The initial signs and symptoms in both are the same for the first 48-72 hours but after this interval the symptoms do not begin to resolve in intramuscular and pain, swelling and loss of move-

DAMAGE TO MUSCLES Section through limb

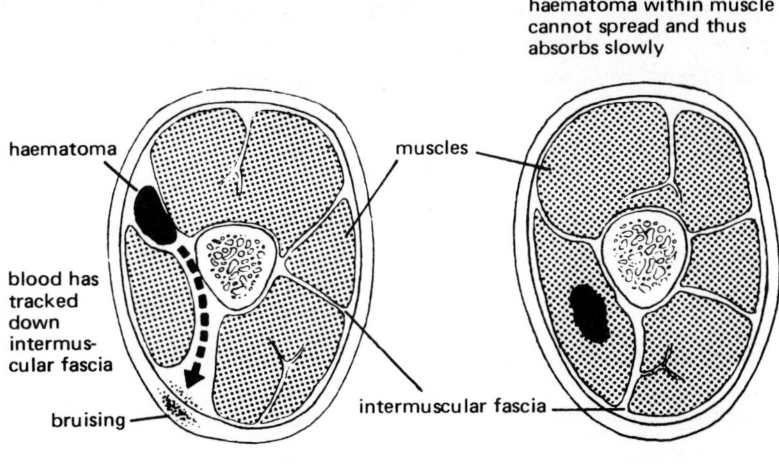

ment are still marked. A tender lump (haematoma) may be felt in the muscles; it can occasionally be aspirated (by doctor who can also give a spreading agent like 'Varidase', or tablets like Chymoral). No physiotherapy or heating should be undertaken (while pain persists), as it will further damage the delicate muscle fibres. Progress is much slower but similar to intERmuscular (usually two or three times longer with intRA-muscular). Recovery from muscle injury has not taken place until FULL POWER, EXTENSIBILITY, RANGE OF JOINT MOVEMENT and SKILL PATTERN have returned. The muscle's ability to stretch to its fullest (extensibility) is vital for maximum power e.g. a high jumper's crouch stretches the necessary muscle groups before the explosive contraction and spring into the air. Without full extensibility athletic performance falls.

c). Muscles may tear at the *musculo-tendinous* or *musculo-periosteal* junctions. Swelling is often minimal but loss of function considerable. Treatment as above, with steroid injections, by doctor. *Tendo-periosteal* tears are managed in the same way, and can occasionally tear off small flakes of bone (torn ligaments sometimes do the same) which may require a plaster of paris for several weeks.

Most common pulled muscles in sportsmen are the hamstrings and quadriceps of the thigh, the origin of sartorius and rectus fermois at the iliac spines, ilio-psoas at the lesser trochanter and the adductor longus on the pubic symphysis.

POSITION OF MUSCLE INJURY (Pulled muscle)

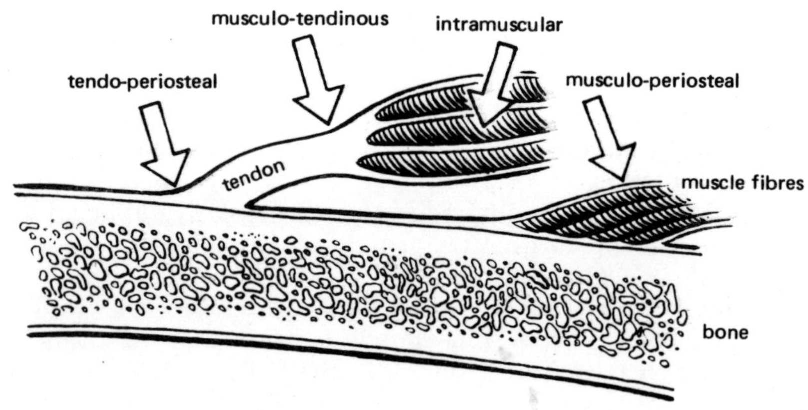

MUSCLE FIBRES CANNOT REGENERATE AND ARE REPLACED BY SCAR TISSUE that weakens the muscles and forms palpable nodules.

RECENT MUSCLE INJURIES (within 48 hours)
CANNOT BE RUN OFF
HEATED AWAY
MASSAGED AWAY
STRETCHED, PULLED OR MANIPULATED AWAY
ELECTRICALLY STIMULATED AWAY
OR INJECTED AWAY.

Anyone attempting such should be sent away, RAPIDLY.

DANGERS OF MUSCLE INJURY
- .... weakness of scar and recurrent tearing,
- .... infection of haematoma,
- .... cyst formation of haematoma,
- .... adhesion of scar to other muscles, bone, or tendon limiting mobility and full extensibility.
- .... myositis ossificans, when the haematoma is converted into bone, which markedly interferes with normal muscle activity.
- .... Such bony lumps are difficult to excise and can ruin an athletic career.

Resting a muscle only leads to atrophy of the fibres, the restoration of full muscle function is an interaction of rest, exercises (static, active and passive) including all muscles and joints in the limb concerned, that needs patience and understanding. NEVER RUSH AN ATHLETE back to full activity before he is competent in training. If he/she breaks down then all confidence is lost.

STIFFNESS is due to an accumulation of oedema in muscles due to unaccustomed or strenuous exercise, and since striated muscle has no lymph vessels, the blood vessels are temporarily unable to cope. The soleus of the calf is a 'sponge' of vessels pumping blood back to the heart (often called the peripheral heart) and is usually the first muscle to suffer.

Treatment: elevation of the limb and gentle massage towards the heart.

STAGES FOLLOWING MUSCLE INJURY

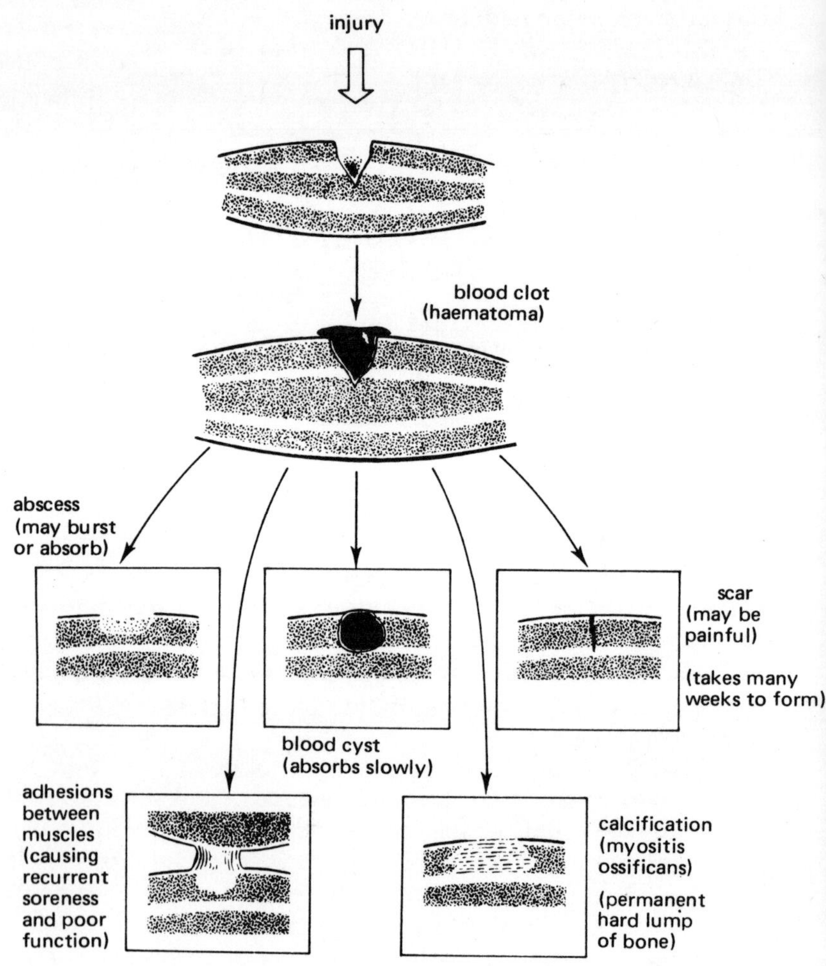

Injuries to the Head

SCALP WOUNDS . . . The scalp consists of four layers of tissues intimately adherent and richly supplied with blood vessels. The scalp usually splits through all layers to the skull and bleeds freely. Because of the vascularity these wounds heal rapidly. A haematoma of the scalp may be subcutaneous or beneath the muscle layer. A BOGGY swelling may overlie a FRACTURE OF THE SKULL.

Treatment: pressure dressing, suturing (Casualty Department etc.).

INJURIES TO THE SKULL BONES . . . A fracture of the skull itself is not important; it is the bleeding beneath the bones and the possible damage to the soft brain substance that matters. May be SIMPLE or COMPOUND. May be LINEAR, COMMINUTED or DEPRESSED.

LINEAR FRACTURES are usually simple and due to compression of the round vault of the skull. Commonly produced by falls against a flat object.

COMMINUTED FRACTURES have several small bony fragments and are more dangerous, since they are caused by short rounded or sharp objects which can drive the pieces into the brain or covering meninges. Often compound.

DEPRESSED FRACTURES are caused by blows from a large rounded object and the scalp is often left intact. Common after kicks on the head in football or rugger.

Diagnosis—by X-ray.

Treatment of simple fractures is by bed rest for three weeks. The other types may require operation depending on the degree of displacement. ALL FRACTURES OF THE SKULL MUST BE EXAMINED FOR POSSIBLE BRAIN INJURY.

Usually the clinical features of a fracture are obvious and commonly the scalp is damaged by the force necessary to fracture the bones. Classically a BOGGY swelling is found and the fracture line may be visible in the wound. Fractures at the temporal region (above the ear) can cause tearing of the middle meningeal

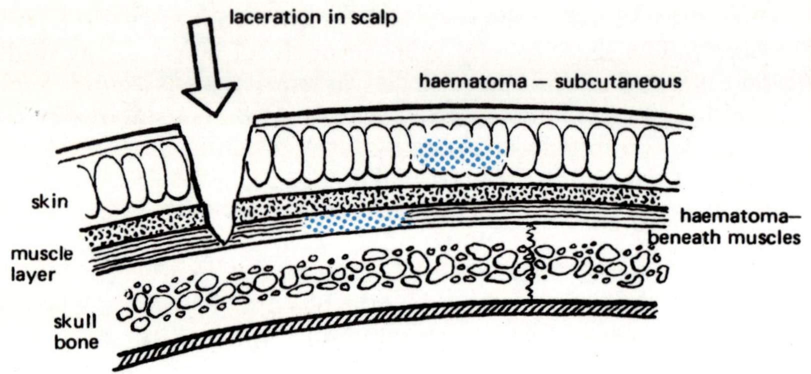
laceration in scalp
haematoma – subcutaneous
skin
haematoma–
beneath muscles
muscle
layer
skull
bone

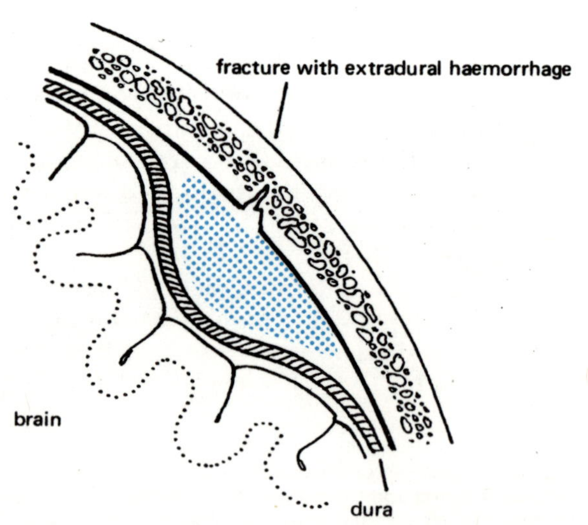
fracture with extradural haemorrhage
brain
dura

artery or vein and an extradural haemorrhage. Fractures above the nose (frontal) region) may break the cribriform plate and allow the escape of cerebrospinal fluid (clear like crystal water or tinged with blood) from the nose. The casualty must on no account blow his nose or air is forced through the fracture and into the skull, with the risk of meningitis. A black eye appearing some hours after a head injury, with no damage to the skin around the eye and with a flame-shaped haemorrhage beneath the conjunctiva, indicates a fracture to the anterior fossa of the skull. Bleeding from the ear, if derived from a torn drum or damaged external meatus, will clot, if mixed with cerebrospinal fluid it continues to drip and indicates a fractured middle fossa. A boggy swelling at the nape of the neck or discoloration behind the mastoid process indicates a fracture to the posterior fossa.

'Contre-coup' injuries—The soft brain moves after the skull when the head is struck and a contre-coup injury is produced e.g. a blow on the forehead knocks the skull backwards and hits the stationary brain on its anterior aspect before the brain tissue begins to move backwards and perhaps damages its posterior lobe against the posterior surface of the skull. Symptoms from such injuries can often be very difficult to evaluate.

Head injuries can be somewhat prevented by protective headgear e.g. in cycling, horseriding.

STAGES IN A FRACTURE OF THE SKULL

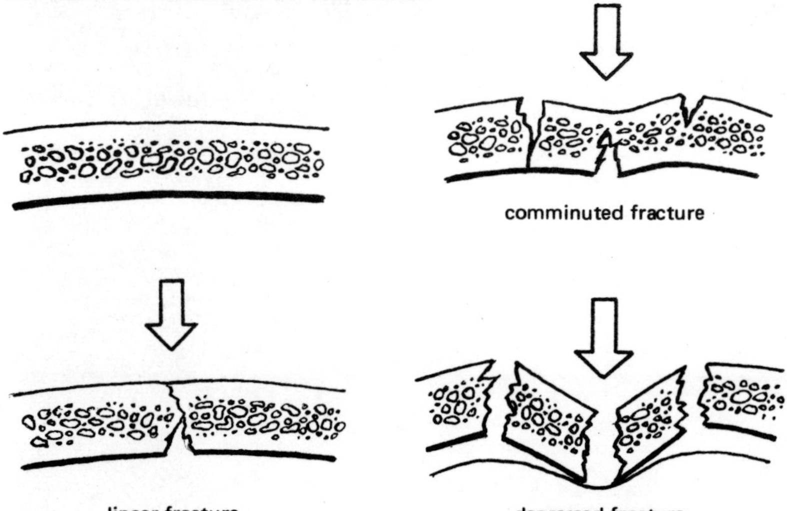

comminuted fracture

linear fracture

depressed fracture

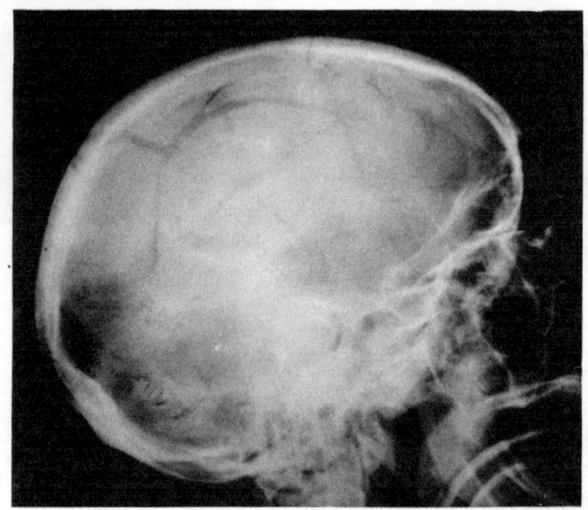

Xray showing
linear fracture

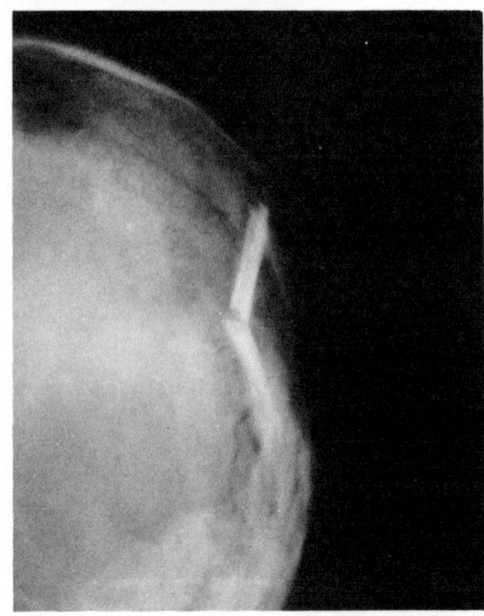

Xray showing
depressed fracture

Injuries to the Brain Substance

Commonly, though not invariably, associated with fractures of the skull. The brain may be injured DIRECTLY or by COMPRESSION from swelling or bleeding within the skull.

ALL DEGREES OF BRAIN INJURY RESULT IN LOSS OF CONSCIOUSNESS, which may be MOMENTARY. CONFUSION, IRRITABILITY or DELIRIUM are found. On recovery the player complains of headache, photophobia and vomiting may ensue. SERIOUS SIGNS are dilated or irregular pupils, irregular respiration, rapid and feeble pulse, and paralysis of face or limbs (see care of the unconscious patient).

THE NECK MAY BE INJURED AT THE SAME TIME, usually by being forced backwards.

TRAUMATIC INTRACRANIAL HAEMORRHAGE is of three types a) subcortical b) extradural and c) subdural.

SUBCORTICAL haemorrhage is produced by arterial bleeding on or in the brain substance and is of a serious nature. Subarachnoid haemorrhage may arise from small and large vessels, so that blood is found in the cerebrospinal fluid. EXTRADURAL haemorrhage results from injury to the middle meningeal vessels (either anterior or posterior). The cause is a laterally directed injury, often relatively trivial, such as a blow from a cricket or golf ball, which strikes the thin plate of the temporal bone. Diagnosis—swelling and bruising in the temporal region (above the ear), a short period of concussion FOLLOWED BY A LUCID PERIOD WHEN THE PLAYER MAY ACT NORMALLY, later becoming confused, irritable and then UNCONSCIOUS as the bleeding accumulates within the skull and compresses the brain. Weakness, twitching and paralysis of a limb or face may follow. The pupils become irregular then dilated.

ALWAYS BEWARE OF A CONFUSED PLAYER IN THE DRESSING ROOM WITH A BRUISE ON THE TEMPORAL REGION.

Even after a slight period of unconsciousness any player must LEAVE the field. Exercise, with its enormous increase in blood flow, will make the potentially lethal bleeding worse.
Treatment: see care of seriously injured. URGENT MEDICAL ADVICE WANTED AT HOSPITAL.
SUBDURAL haemorrhage is produced by rupture of the veins passing from the brain to the venous sinuses on the inside of the dural covering of the skull. Usually produced by blows of small amplitude applied to the front or back of the head which may occasionally be insufficient to produce unconsciousness. Diagnosis—as above, but usually no skull fracture evident.
Treatment: as above.

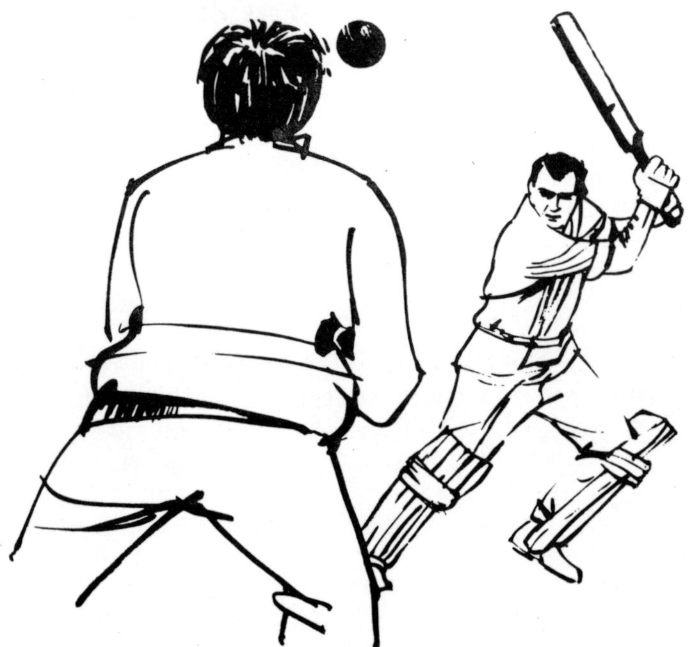

Blow on temporal region—common cause of head injuries

SUB-DURAL HAEMORRGAGE

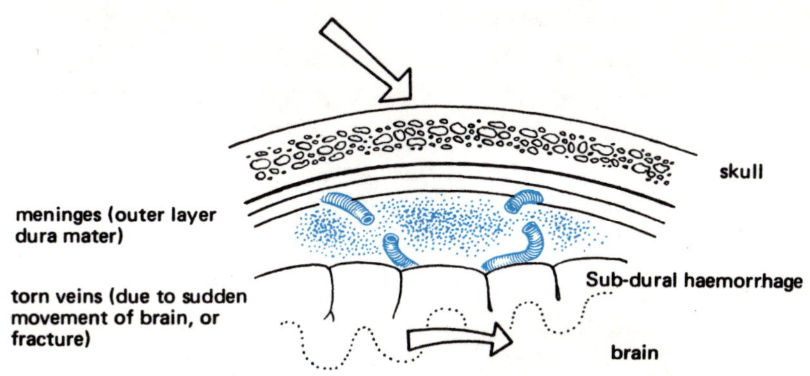

EXTRADURAL HAEMORRHAGE

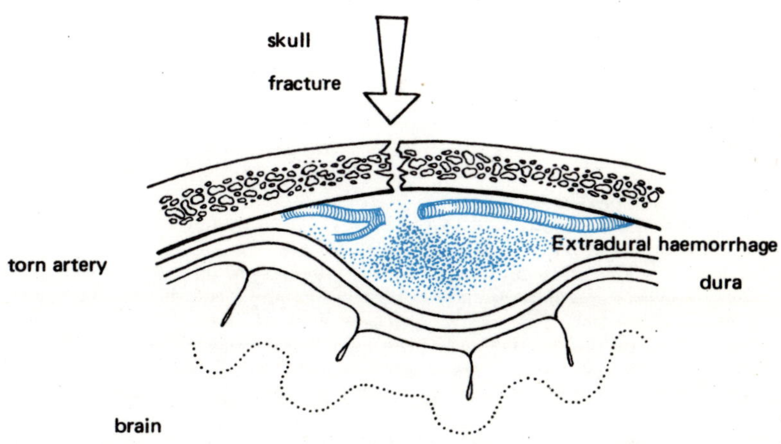

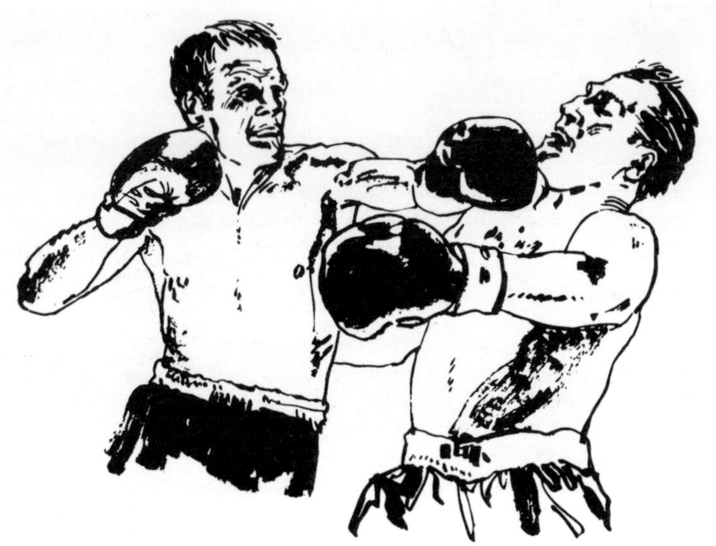

Boxing—repeated trauma to face, and chest.
Concussion caused by direct blow or accumulation of effects. (see text)

Concussion in **boxing** is caused by a direct blow to the lower jaw, by an accumulation of the effects of blows on the head, or by the head striking the floor of the ring. Unconsciousness may also be produced by a blow on the carotid sinus in the neck, over the heart, or to the solar plexus (although in the latter case the boxer often remains conscious throughout, but is unable to rise due to a temporary paralysis of his legs. This paralysis subsides with no ill effects.) If consciousness has not been regained by the end of the count the boxer is allowed to recover on the floor of the ring, in the semiprone position. The punch drunk syndrome is almost non-existent in amateur boxers, but found in some professionals of the 'slugger' variety.
In sports liable to head injuries, e.g. cycle racing, rock climbing, horse riding, etc. a protective helmet MUST be worn.

Injuries to the Face

Lacerations on the eyebrows need rapid compression with a cold sponge to prevent a black eye. Dumb-bell sutures usually suffice. Cut lips, crossing the vermilion (red portion) on to the face, need suture and close approximation of the parts to prevent deformity. Haematomas on the ear need aspiration or incision to allow the clot to escape and prevent the formation of a cauliflower ear, followed by a pressure dressing. The ear drum is occasionally injured in diving, with immediate pain, buzzing, varying degree of deafness on that side.

CORNEAL ABRASIONS often resemble foreign bodies in the eye. They can only be diagnosed by a dye technique in hospital. Foreign bodies are removed with clean cotton pad or lavage with warm water. They often escape under the UPPER LID, which should be everted over a matchstick.

LOSS of vision after a blow on the eye, as in boxing, may be due to a DETACHED RETINA or VITREOUS HAEMORRHAGE. Requires urgent admission to casualty department.

The NASAL BONES are commonly fractured in all contact sports, especially boxing. Can be reduced at once or when the swelling subsides (approximately 4+ days). DISPLACEMENT OF THE CARTILAGES is equally as common and the deformity usually obvious. Treat as fracture. Boxing can be resumed after 2–3 months.

EPISTAXIS can be combatted by gently pinching the nose and applying pressure with a cold sponge. Nasal packing with adrenaline solutions may be necessary. Bleeding from the nose may indicate a fractured nasal bone, or a displaced septum which may require manipulation in Casualty Dept.

FRACTURES OF THE MAXILLA are usually the result of a direct blow, and may involve the upper teeth. Treatment is usually by rest and mouth washes, but a dental splint may be needed.

FRACTURES OF THE MALAR (or ZYGOMATIC) BONE occur during a corner at soccer when there is a clash of heads. Diagnosis—flattening of the cheek, numbness of the face, difficulty in opening the mouth and double vision.

Treatment: elevation by surgical means if seriously depressed.

FRACTURES OF THE MANDIBLE are caused by blows on the chin or side of the face, common in boxing.

Diagnosis—pain, difficulty in speaking and swallowing, blood-stained saliva and irregularity in the line of the teeth.

Treatment: supportive bandage (see p. 7). Refer to dental department.

Fractures of the neck of the condyle, coronoid process, and ascending ramus are well splinted by the powerful muscles

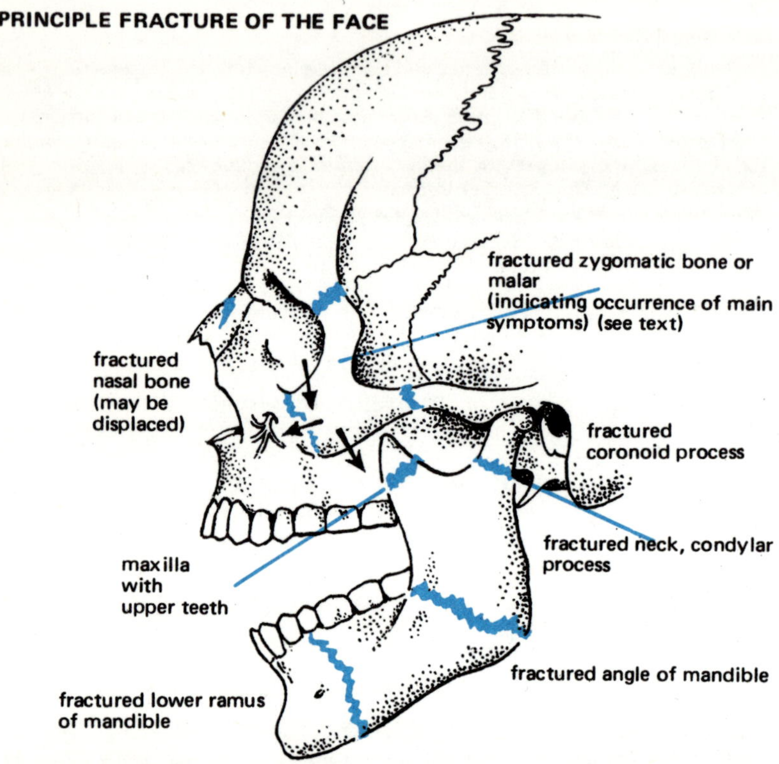

that surround them. Fractures of the horizontal ramus need dental splinting with wires etc. Activity can be resumed in 3–4 months, except boxing (6 months).

DISLOCATION OF THE MANDIBLE due to a blow on the chin when the mouth is partly open. Diagnosis—the lower jaw is displaced to one side (unless bilateral), saliva dribbles down the chin, and a hollow is felt in front of the ear.

Treatment: reduction can be performed by pressing the padded thumbs on the lower molar teeth, rotating the chin inwards and upwards with the fingers. Occasionally an anaesthetic is needed. A support is worn for 2–4 weeks.

Injuries to the Spine

The spine is a segmented lever of 33 small bones connected by strong ligaments and muscles protecting the spinal cord and nerves. Backache may indicate bony, or ligamentous damage.

SPRAINS are common and muscle fibres are occasionally torn while lifting heavy weights (weight lifting, hammer or javelin throwing, high and long jumping) or a sudden movement in a match. Pain is usually localised and a tender spot found. Young tennis players with a poor serve often develop backstrain, and occasionally a scoliosis (bending) of the spine, which may also be found in 'one sided' oarsmen.

Treatment: rest, analgesics (aspirin etc.), heat.

FRACTURES OF THE SPINE. INCOMPLETE FRACTURES involve the spinous processes, transverse processes, lamina and compression fractures of the vertebral body. COMPLETE FRACTURES interrupt the continuity of the spinal column and are called fracture-dislocations. These may occur at any level and are found in riding accidents. Complete fractures commonly occur at the points of maximum mobility, C.5 to C.7 and L.3 to L.5, or at the junction of fixed and mobile portions, especially the thoracic/lumbar junction. Separation commonly occurs through a disc.

Treatment: Incomplete fractures heal after 3-6 weeks bed rest or P.O.P. Complete fractures may need P.O.P.; or surgical reduction and fixation, with hospitalisation for 2-3 months.

In all fractures of the spine DAMAGE TO THE SPINAL CORD IS THE MOST IMPORTANT FACTOR. Diagnosis—sudden severe pain over the spine, may radiate round to the front of the body, inability to move, numbness and weakness. The immediate effect of the injury produces spinal shock with a flaccid paralysis below the damaged area, with loss of sensation. The stage of spinal shock lasts for 48 hours or longer and as the swelling decreases the recovery of nervous activity may be noted.

FRACTURES OF THE CERVICAL SPINE. Since the cervical region is highly mobile, fracture-dislocation can occur with relatively minor forces sustained during sports exercise e.g. falls on the head in riding, diving, football and rugger. Cord damage is rarer than in other regions because the cord is smaller here in relationship to the bony arch that surrounds it.

FRACTURES OF THE THORACIC (DORSAL) SPINE. This region has strength but little mobility and is usually only

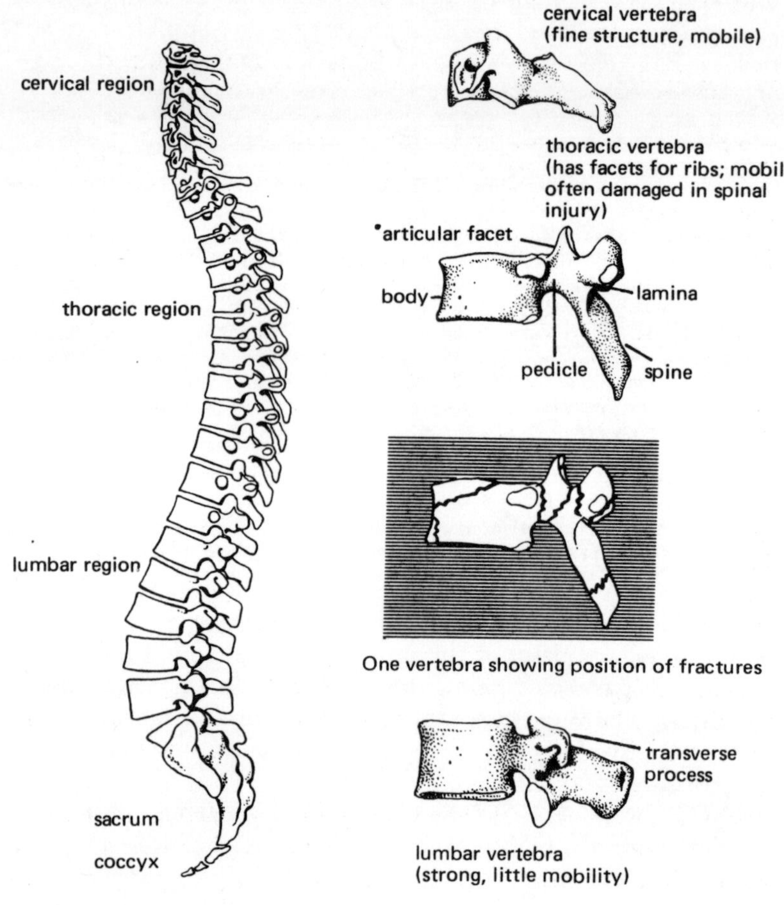

Illustration of spinal bones (connecting ligaments not shown). Spinal cord within collumn of bones

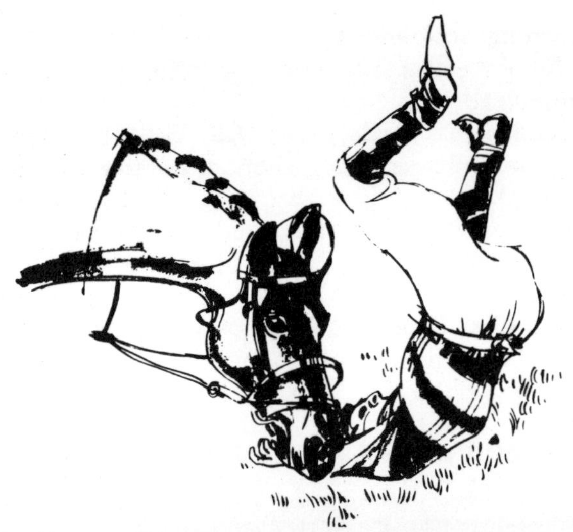

Horse riders are prone to injuries of clavicle, shoulder, and spinal bones. This incident shows the cervical region taking the impact.

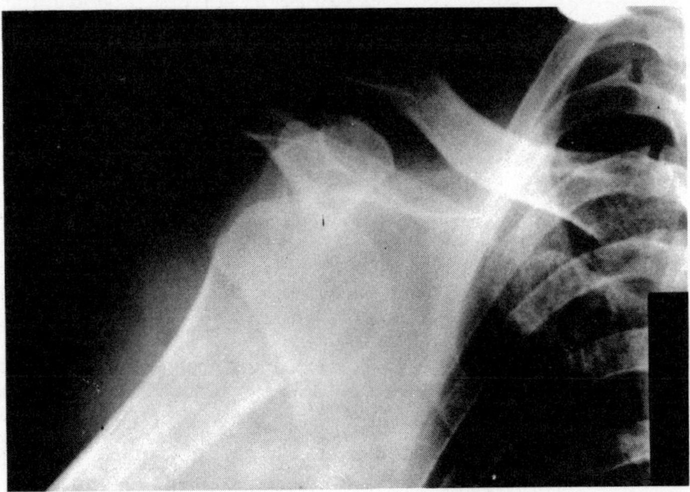

Xray showing dislocation (anterior) of humeral head, which now lies away from the glenoid cavity at the lateral edge of the scapula.

injured in riding accidents e.g. the curved back of the jockey taking the full force of a fall. When the injury is severe the cord is usually damaged.

FRACTURES OF THE LUMBAR SPINE. Here great strength and mobility exist together. A relatively major force is required to produce injury. Below L.2–L.3 the spinal cord does not exist and the vertebral canal is occupied with nerve roots which are rarely injured.

FRACTURES OF THE SACRUM are rare, but strain of the posterior sacro-iliac ligaments commonly produces a dull ache at the base of the spine, 2″ from the midline.

FRACTURES OF THE COCCYX are uncommon and require little treatment.

PROLAPSE OF AN INTERVERTEBRAL DISC is only found in persons whose discs already show degeneration. May occur in weight lifters and gymnasts. Sciatica may accompany any such disorder. Wrestlers are prone to cervical disc troubles, while high divers may injure the lumbar discs.

Treatment: by rest, heat and analgesics, and physiotherapy.

COMPRESSION FRACTURES of a vertebral body cause wedging of the bone, usually the anterior aspect.

Treatment: by rest (3–4 weeks) in bed or plaster jacket. Pain and deformity of the spine lead to diagnosis.

TRUE DISLOCATIONS (WITHOUT FRACTURE) only commonly occur in the cervical spine, usually C.5/6, C.6/7. Need reduction immediately in hospital.

Back-ache may be due to congenital bony abnormalities or bony conditions like spondylolisthesis, when one vertebral body slips forward on another. X-ray diagnosis. May need simple lumbar support, physiotherapy or operation.

Horse riders, especially **steeple-chase jockeys** are prone to injuries to the spinal bones, the most common cause of injury is when the horse stumbles or falls on landing from a jump, the rider being pitched forward. This cause accounts for 80–85% of the injuries situated above the waist, a fractured clavicle or dislocated acromio-clavicular joint and dislocated shoulder being most usual as it is this region that hits the ground first. Landing on the face may injure the cervical spine by hyperextension, landing on a curved back may injure the lumbar and thoracic. When the horse rolls over the rider the ribs, pelvis and thigh are at risk. Helmets should be worn to protect the head. Occasionally a rider loses his position and he may fall forward striking his face against the horse's neck. Serious accidents can often be avoided by falling away from the horse, releasing the reins to effect clean separation.

INJURIES TO CLAVICLE

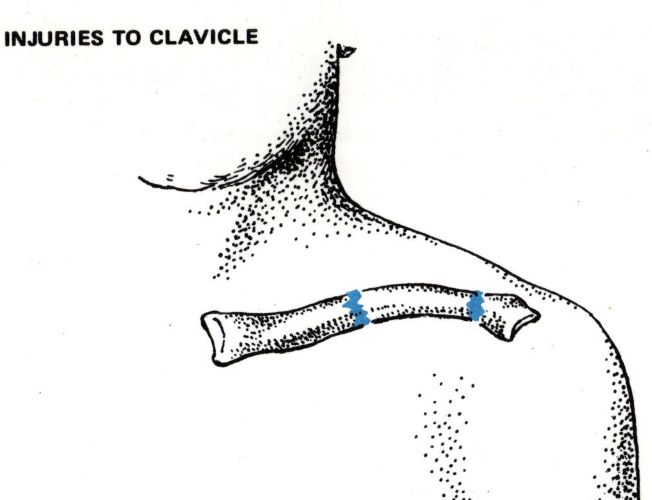

Illustration showing two common sites for fractures of the clavicle

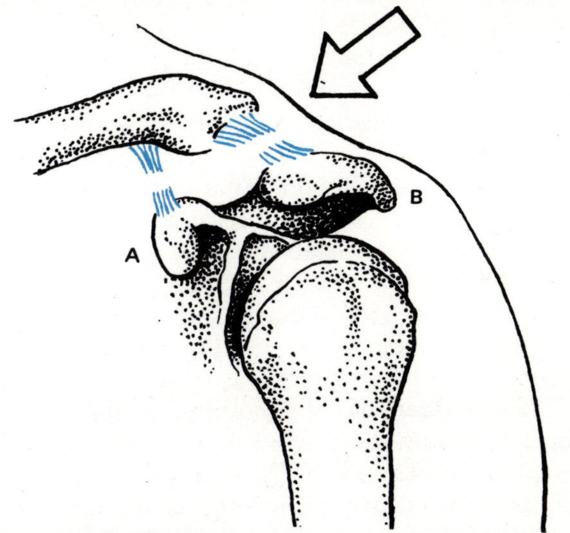

Illustration showing dislocation of the clavicle from the coracoid process (A) and acromion process (B) of the scapula

Injuries to the Clavicle etc.

These injuries are common in soccer, rugby football and amongst jockeys, but in American football padded shoulders are used for protection.

FRACTURE. The clavicle is the commonest long bone to fracture, usually due to a fall on to an outstretched hand. Since this bone lies just under the skin diagnosis is easy for the deformity can be seen and palpated.

Treatment: a figure of 8 bandage for 3 or more weeks. Rapid return to sports activities.

DISLOCATION. Occasionally the inner (sternal) end of the clavicle is dislocated; pain, deformity and abnormal position are obvious. Rarely it presses onto the trachea from gross upward displacement over the sternal notch.

Treatment: strapping in position and sling for 6 weeks. May not hold and operation needed.

Disloction of the ACROMIOCLAVICULAR JOINT is common after a fall onto the shoulder following a heavy tackle at soccer or rugger, and in high jumping. The outer end of the clavicle is forced up and overrides the acromium of the scapula. A prominence is felt over the shoulder.

Treatment: The forearm is flexed and 'Elastoplast' bandage is applied around the elbow and over a felt pad situated across the reduced dislocation, at the outer end of the clavicle. The arm is then supported with a sling for 3–6 weeks. Surgery and internal fixation may be needed.

FRACTURES OF THE SCAPULA. Because this bone is well covered with muscles, swelling and bruising are limited by their sheaths, and treatment is by a sling for 3 or more weeks. Shoulder movements are painful with this type of injury and occasionally an erroneous diagnosis of a shoulder injury is made. Breathing may be painful and possible fractured rib(s) lying beneath the scapula MUST be excluded.

In the above injuries, while the sling is being worn, the fingers, forearm and arm muscles should be exercised with either active or static contractions. IN ALL CASES OF LIMB IMMOBI-

LISATION MENTIONED HEREAFTER ONLY THE NECESSARY PARTS SHOULD REMAIN AT REST, ALL OTHERS SHOULD BE LIGHTLY EXERCISED TO MAINTAIN TONE AND MOBILITY AND THUS SPEED RECOVERY.

The BRACHIAL PLEXUS may be damaged when the angle between the shoulder and the neck is opened out by a fall at speed—speedway rider, huntsman—and the delicate nerve roots stretched at their point of origin from the spinal cord or in the posterior triangle of the neck. Treatment is by rest and physiotherapy, with operative repair of torn nerves (see Shoulder injuries and Arm).

BASEBALL PLAYERS often develop marked discomfort in the scapular region due to irritation of the suprascapula nerve by hard throwing. They also develop degeneration in the supraspinatus, bicipital tendinitis, and acute and chronic bursitis of the subacromial bursa. Occasionally they accumulate calcium deposits in the long head of triceps, just below the shoulder joint, which presents with severe pain on throwing. An X-ray will aid diagnosis (see add. longus). They also commonly injure the elbow, and olecranon fractures are not uncommon. Finger injuries (mallet finger) are often found.

SHOULDER INJURIES

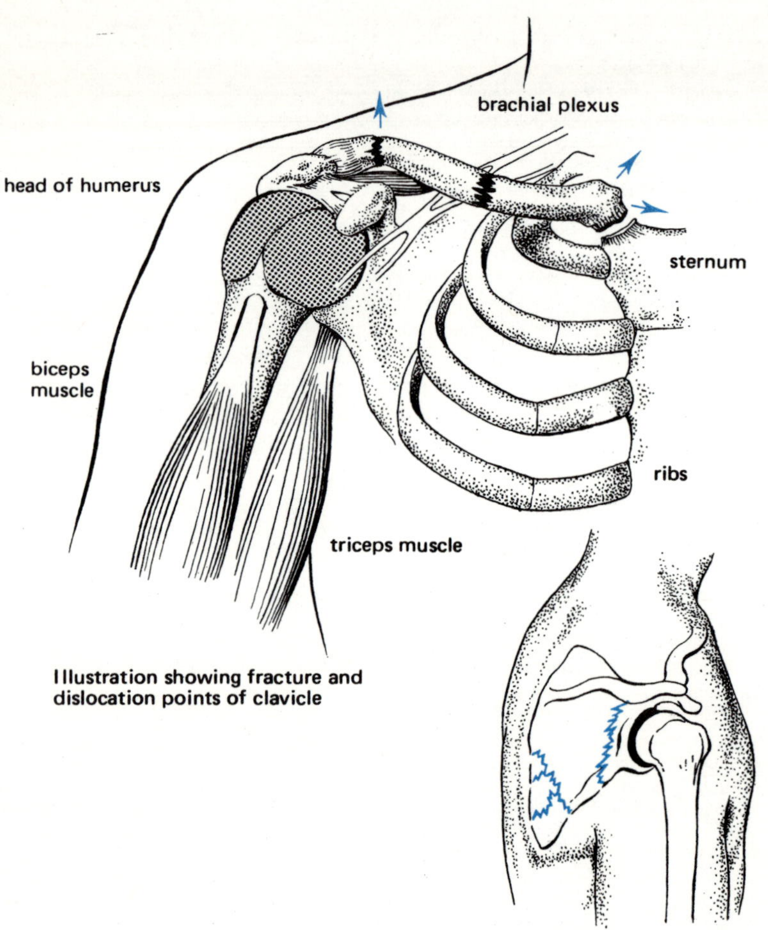

Illustration showing fracture and dislocation points of clavicle

Illustration showing fractures of body of scapula

Injury to the Shoulder

The cup of the glenoid cavity of the scapula is shallow and the humeral head enjoys an enormous range of movement. Thus the ligaments of the shoulder are reinforced by small muscles (rotator cuff) which have become part of the capsule of the joint. The deltoid is the bulky ensheathing muscle and any damage, e.g. bruising and swelling, occurs beneath it.

DISLOCATION . . . is common in high jumpers, water polo players, collision at swimming and throwing events, but can occur when any player falls on to an outstretched arm or shoulder so that the humerus is forcibly abducted and laterally rotated. Then the head slips out of the lower aspect of the glenoid cavity and passes *anteriorly* where it forms a prominent elevation under the coracoid process. The normal rounded outline of the shoulder is lost. There is a sickly pain, muscle spasm and the patient supports the limb with the other hand. Occasionally numbness is found around the upper arm due to a crushing of the circumflex (axillary) nerve. Sometimes the head passes POSTERIORLY and the rounded outline of the shoulder is maintained. Pain is severe and movements restricted. Special X-rays are needed for this rare type.

Treatment: support with a sling, reduction is carried out in hospital with or without an anaesthetic, depending on spasm. DO NOT REDUCE A DISLOCATION ON THE FIELD UNLESS IT IS VERY RECURRENT. A FRACTURE MAY COEXIST AND AN ATTEMPTED REDUCTION CAN DAMAGE THE IMPORTANT NERVES AND ARTERIES OF THE AXILLA.

Do not forget that for a dislocation to occur the ligaments, muscles and joint capsule must be stretched or torn. Even after prompt reduction persisting weakness may be found, with the formation of a stiff or frozen shoulder. Damage to the SUPRASPINATUS tendon, which stabilises the humeral head for the deltoid to act, leads to an inability to abduct the arm during the first 15–20° of movement. If the limb is supported through this stage then the deltoid takes over and full abduction follows. Rupture needs surgical suture.

RECURRENT DISLOCATIONS require operative treatment and are prone to occur during the 'hand off' at rugger or in the high jump in the overbalance stage of the roll.

FROZEN SHOULDER may arise out of the blue, after injections, illness or injury in the shoulder or arm. ALL ranges of movement are severely limited. Heat, physiotherapy, anti-inflammatory tablets and steroid injections are used. Until full recovery, which may take months, the full swing of the golfer or tennis smash is limited.

CALCIFICATION AND DEGENERATION in the small muscles and tendons around the joint is sometimes found in athletes (especially swimmers), the SUPRASPINATUS is often implicated as supraspinatus tendinitis when pain is produced with 50+ of abduction at the shoulder. An accompanying swelling of the subacromial bursa may occur, and a tender spot deep to the deltoid at the tip of the acromial end of the clavicle is found. These troubles are common in spin bowlers when accurate controlling action of the deltoid puts considerable pressure on the subjacent bursa, and in tennis and golf. An X-ray occasionally shows calcification. Treatment: heat, ultrasound, physiotherapy, anti-inflammatory tablets and steroid injections.

PAIN over the shoulder may be referred from the neck as a form of brachial neuralgia, treatment of the underlying cervical condition is required.

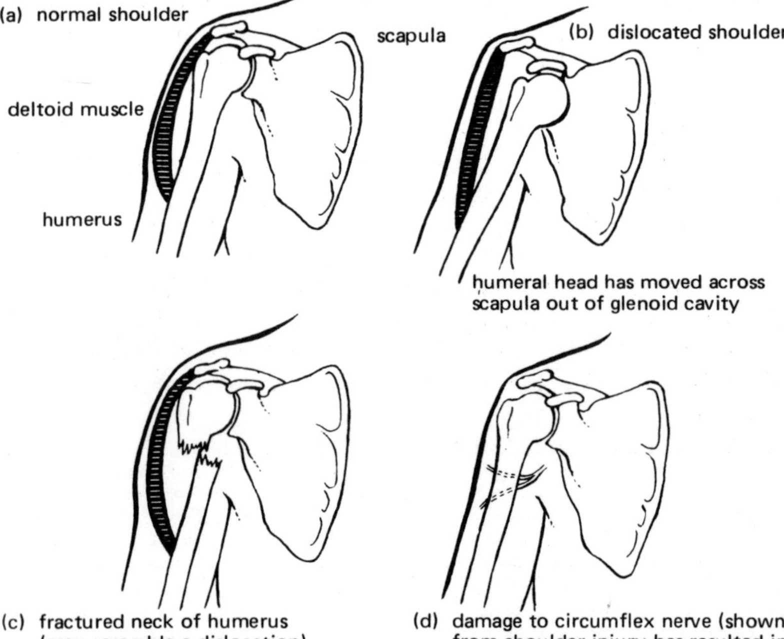

(c) fractured neck of humerus (may resemble a dislocation) (see text)

(d) damage to circumflex nerve (shown) from shoulder injury has resulted in flattening of shoulder and loss of deltoid muscle

SHOULDER MUSCLE INJURY

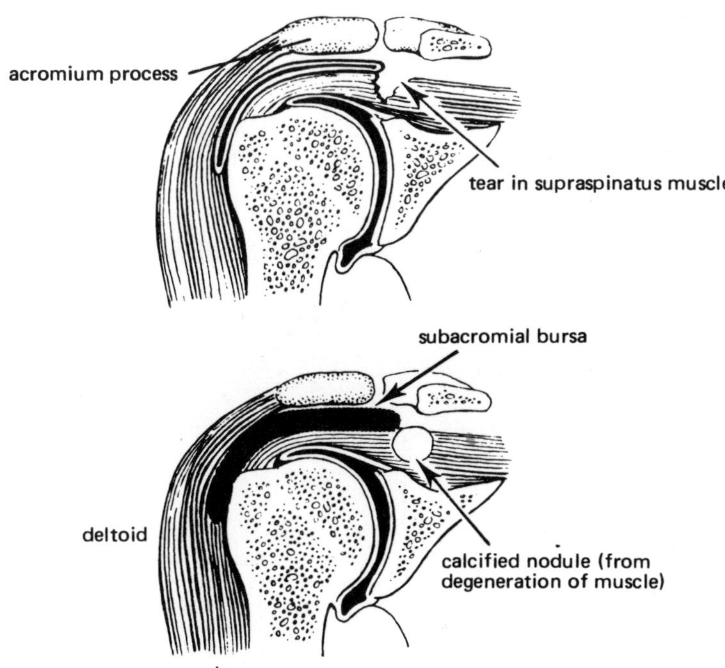

calcified nodule in supraspinatus muscle, has caused—by friction—a swelling of the subacromial bursa

FRACTURES OF THE HUMERUS

Illustration showing position of humerus and radial nerve in arm

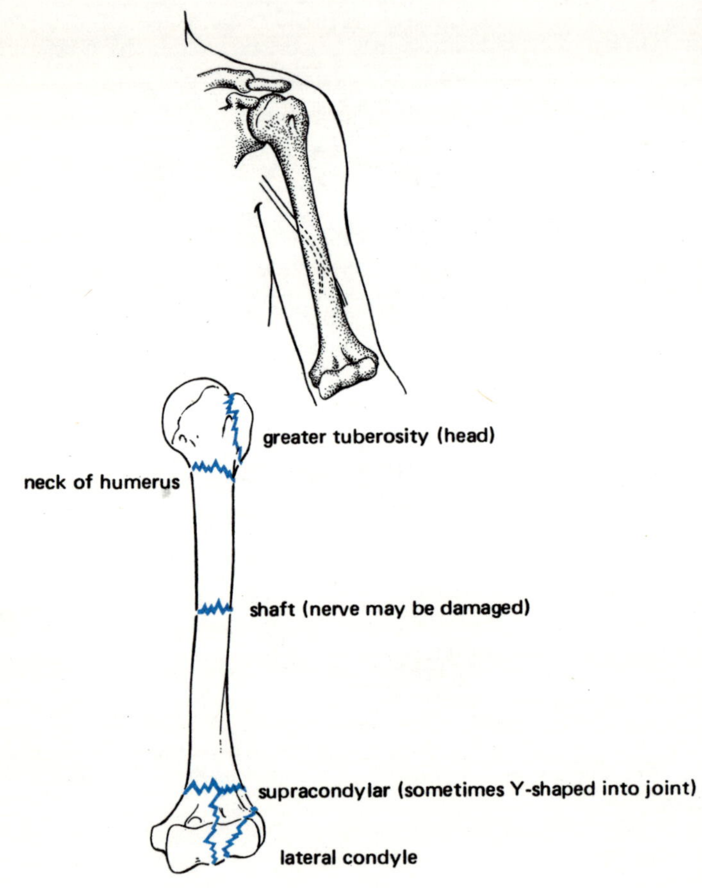

Injury to the Arm

TENDINITIS OF THE BICEPS TENDON follows unaccustomed use such as vigorous tennis or golf (often called golfer's shoulder). The shoulder looks normal but tenderness is found in the bicipital groove and on external rotation.
Treatment: rest and local heat, local anaesthetic injections and deep frictions.
RUPTURE OF THE BICEPS may be found after severe exertion especially with age. Diagnosis is unmistakable for the belly of the muscle is too low and looks plump instead of the normal elongation, and it does not tighten on movement.
Treatment: in the elderly none, in the younger person suture may be needed.
BRACHIAL NEURALGIA is a vague term applied to pain extending over a large part of the upper limb. May be due to a fall on the neck or shoulder and minor damage to the nerve roots, to mild osteoarthritis or disc degeneration in the cervical spine or to rheumatoid degeneration in the capsule of the shoulder.
Treatment: rest, perhaps with a collar for the neck, heat, physiotherapy and manipulation, analgesics and anti-inflammatory agents.
PROLAPSED CERVICAL DISC. The factors responsible are the same as those of lumbar disc prolapse, usually sudden unguarded movements in degenerating discs. Pain and stiffness is observed, with radiation of pain to the shoulder and scapular region (fibrositis). Pins and needles, numbness and occasional weakness are found in the upper limb. Between attacks of mild disc trouble the patient feels well. An attack may begin suddenly with acute torticollis (wry neck).
Treatment: analgesics, muscle relaxants, rest in a collar, heat, traction and physiotherapy.

FRACTURES OF THE HUMERUS.

NECK . . . from a fall on the outstretched hand. Extensive bruising of the arm with a painful shoulder, and may resemble a dislocation.
Treatment: no reduction unless displaced. Collar and cuff, 3–6 weeks.

GREATER TUBEROSITY. From direct blows. Symptoms and signs are for a fracture but tenderness is felt beneath the covering deltoid muscle at the tip of the shoulder and abduction is severely limited.
Treatment: undisplaced fractures need sling for 3–6 weeks, but displaced fractures, due to muscle pull require special operative or supportive treatment i.e. an abduction frame for 6–12 weeks.
SHAFT occurs after a fall on to the hand that twists the humerus causing a spiral fracture, while a fall on to the elbow produces an oblique or transverse fracture. Diagnosis is easy due to gross deformity, swelling and loss of function.
Treatment: Collar and cuff or plaster of paris (P.O.P.) U-slab for 4–8 weeks.

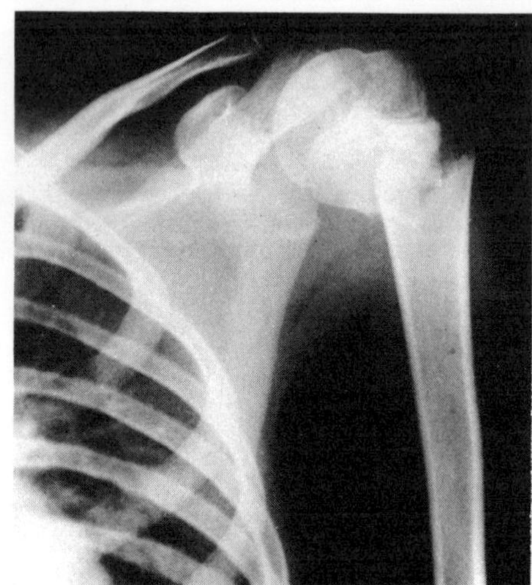

Xray showing fractured neck of humerus

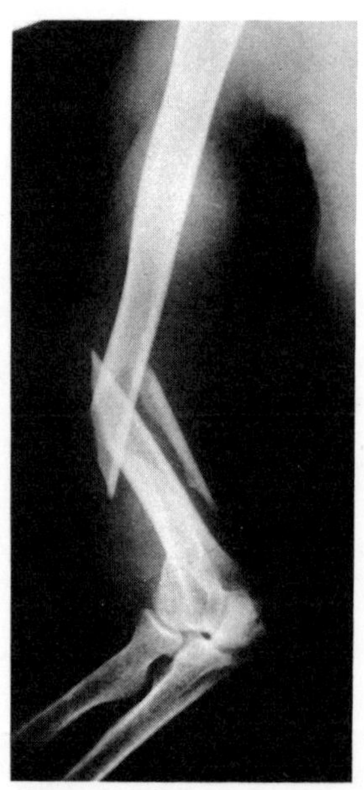

Xray showing fractured shaft of humerus

The Radial nerve runs round the shaft of the humerus and may be damaged with shaft fractures. Sensation on the back of the thumb and forearm, and dorsiflexion of the wrist must be tested (i.e. wrist drop occurs with injury).

Golfers are prone to strains and stiffness in the cervical and lumbar spine. Often there is an underlying pathology like mild osteoarthritis, chronic disc degeneration or some minor bony abnormality. The great strain taken on the wrists and forearms in controlling and adjusting the swing at the moment of impact often produces stiffness and minor tears in the muscle bellies, especially at the origin of the forearm flexors on the medial epicondyle of the elbow (golfer's elbow). Considerable lateral and rotational strain may be placed on the knee joints, especially when playing from an awkward lie with the feet at different levels, and strains of the medial ligament and occasional meniscal damage are found.

SUPRACONDYLAR FRACTURE. THIS IS ONE OF THE MOST SERIOUS FRACTURES and is almost always found in CHILDREN. PERMANENT NERVE, ARTERY AND MUSCLE DAMAGE MAY ENSUE in the forearm if the treatment is NOT PROMPT. Commonly caused by a fall on the hand with the elbow bent, the humerus breaks just above the condyles. The lower fragment, with the forearm, is pushed backwards and twisted inwards. After injury the child holds his forearm with his hand; pain, swelling and deformity are obvious, the BACKWARD SHIFT ABOVE THE ELBOW IS APPARENT. Feel the RADIAL PULSE at the wrist and WATCH THE CIRCULATION for the brachial artery supplying the forearm is often nipped between the bones ends, and goes into spasm or thromboses.

Treatment: TAKE TO HOSPITAL AT ONCE where reduction under general anaesthetic is performed (do not forget the golden rule regarding no drinks or food before anaesthetic). The patient needs observation for 1–2 days in hospital to avoid vascular damage. As the swelling subsides a high/collar and cuff is worn for 3 weeks and gentle movements begun.

Complications: a wasting of the muscles of the forearm may develop if the muscle tissue or nerves are rendered ischaemic from vascular involvement. This condition is known as VOLKMANN'S CONTRACTURE. Joint stiffness at the elbow,

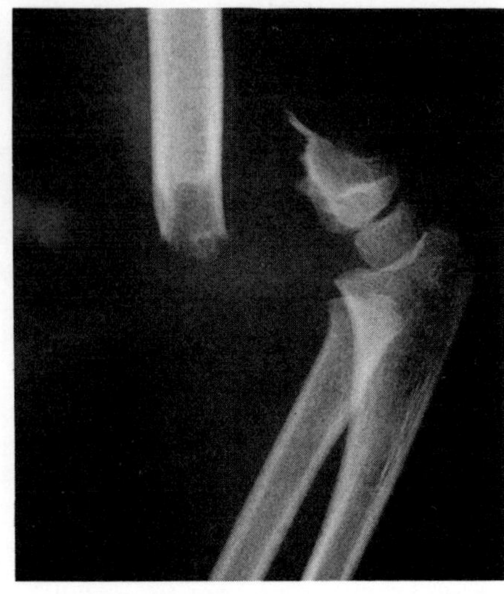

Xray showing supracondylar fracture

and calcification in the muscles (MYOSITIS OSSIFICANS) are also occasionally found.

When the child falls with the elbow STRAIGHT the humerus breaks above the epiphyseal plate and the lower fragment may be tilted forwards (FORWARD DISPLACEMENT OF SUPRACONDYLAR). This injury is uncommon. Treatment: plaster slab with elbow straight for 3 weeks.

T-SHAPED or Y-SHAPED FRACTURES are found at the lower end of the humerus in adults, from a fall on to the point of the elbow. Pain and swelling variable.

Treatment: plaster slab for 6 weeks.

FRACTURE-SEPARATION OF THE LATERAL/MEDIAL CONDYLAR EPIPHYSIS follows a fall onto the elbow in a child. The displacement is usually slight. These injuries need accurate reduction and perhaps operative fixation because a failure in union of the epiphysis with the main shaft of the bone may lead to a warping of the forearm at the elbow due to a cessation of growth at the damaged epiphysis.

Treatment: as described, POP 3-6 weeks.

FRACTURES OF THE CAPITELLUM OR TROCHLEA also need accurate reduction or limited flexion of the elbow results. Surgical intervention may be required with POP for 3–6 weeks. All fractures around the elbow may eventually produce some loss of movement depending upon the degree of damage to the bones and cartilage, and the bleeding into the joint from the damaged capsule and synovial membrane.

Injuries at the Elbow

DISLOCATION: a fall on the hand may dislocate the elbow with resulting deformity and swelling that are obvious; the olecranon is readily felt out of its normal position. Damage to the vessels and nerves may coexist, feel for PULSE and TEST SENSATION. The ULNAR NERVE runs behind the medial epicondyle of the humerus and is the nerve most commonly involved with a dislocation (see nerve injury).

Treatment: reduction under general anaesthetic. First aid measure is gentle but firm splinting in a sling. A collar and cuff is worn for 3 weeks and early movements begun as the swelling subsides.

FRACTURED HEAD OF RADIUS is produced by a fall onto the outstretched hand that forces the forearm into the valgus (extreme lateral) position so that the radial head is knocked against the lower end of the humerus (capitellum), splitting the radial head or breaking a piece off. At the same time the cartilage on the capitellum is damaged and may chip and form a loose body in the elbow joint. After such an injury painful rotation of the forearm is found with localised tenderness over the radial head (1–3 cms) below the lateral epicondyle of the humerus.

Treatment: sling or collar/cuff for three weeks. Severe damage may need excision of the radial head.

FRACTURE OF THE OLECRANON . . . is caused by a fall on to the point of the elbow, or by excessive action of the triceps muscle as in throwing the javelin. Tenderness is easily palpated, with an occasional gap found.

Treatment: sling, or if separation of the bone fragment is seen, screw fixation (or wire).

DISLOCATION OF THE RADIAL HEAD may be part of a fracture of the upper third of the ulna (MONTEGGIA FRACTURE), or rarely on its own.

Treatment: P.O.P. for 12 weeks.

TENNIS ELBOW is common after excessive use of the elbow, classically from repeated backhands at tennis or during the final impetus in javelin or discus throwing. Multiple small tears or chronic inflammation around the origin of the EXTENSOR tendons (of the fingers) produces a dull ache with weakness of dorsiflexion of the hand and a poor grip. A tender spot is found over the lateral epicondyle where these tendons originate, and a handshake with the manipulation of the hand towards the ulna causes pain.

Treatment: rest (may need P.O.P.), heat, alteration in playing technique, ultrasound and steroid injections are used. Rarely operative release of the tendons is performed.

In TENNIS PLAYERS tennis elbow shows itself by pain on the inner or outer aspect of the elbow accentuated by shots on the back hand and the high-kicking service. Sliced strokes, especially the wide, low volley with the backhand are very painful. Pain on the inner side of the elbow is associated with the forehand drive (particularly if top spin is used), the smash and the hard service. Proper warming up, with as much rest as possible when symptoms first appear can do a lot to prevent the condition becoming chronic.

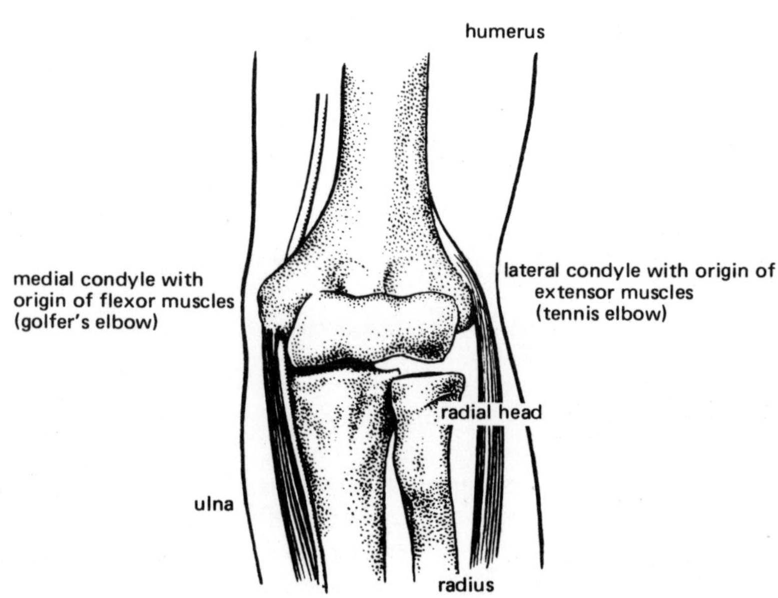

Illustration of elbow joint

INJURIES AT ELBOW

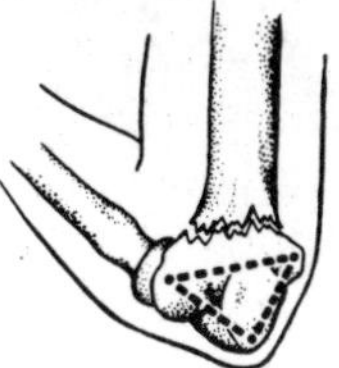

Illustration showing supracondylar fracture (bony points shown by △ can be felt)

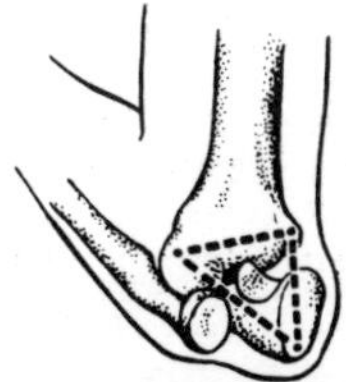

Illustration showing dislocation of elbow (and posterior movement of tip of elbow)

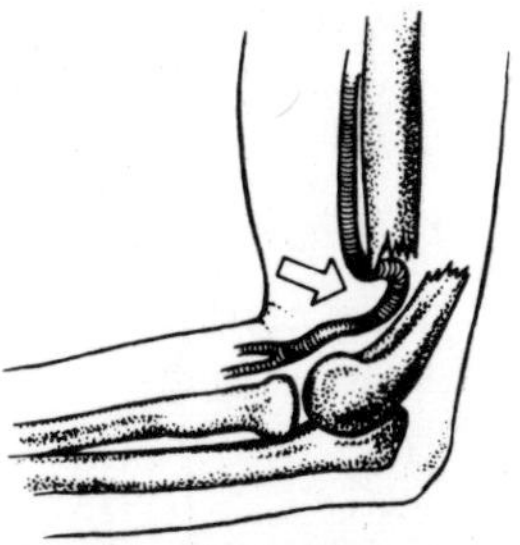

Illustration showing crushing of brachial artery by supracondylar fracture

fractured medial condyle

fractured lateral condyle

fractured capitellum

fractured trochlea

GOLFER'S ELBOW is due to taking too big a divot in the chip shots or by a poor grip that strains the medial ligament of the elbow or the common FLEXOR origin to the fingers. Diagnosis is similar to tennis elbow, except the signs are reversed.

Treatment: as tennis elbow.

BASEBALL ELBOW is a pitcher's injury due to excessive throwing and ultimate swelling of the muscles within the fascia on the anterior aspect of the elbow. A similar condition is found in fast bowlers (away swing action) and in tennis players with a heavily sliced service action.

Treatment: rapidly settles with rest in a sling and elevation.

OSTEOCHONDRITIS DISSECANS may be found in the elbow, and the small fragment of bone which has undergone avascular necrosis may separate and cause locking (see knee).

Javelin Elbow is a painful lesion in the triceps insertion due to minute tears. Sometimes seen in baseball pitchers.

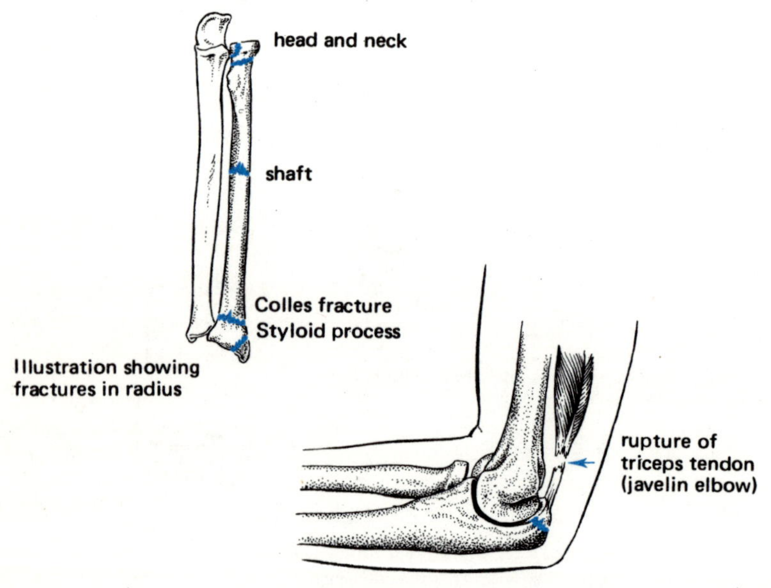

Illustration showing fractures in radius

Illustration showing inner aspect of elbow

Injuries to the Forearm

The two main bones of the forearm, the radius and ulna may be *fractured* individually or together. In single fractures, which are relatively uncommon, the upper or lower radio-ulnar joint is usually damaged. Direct blows are the principle cause. There may be only slight deformity but movements of the bones by gently turning the hand are very painful and it is better to avoid any extra damage by keeping the limb strictly at rest. Since they are relatively superficial, fractures can be detected by running the finger tip along the bony surface and detecting tenderness or deformity.

Treatment: if no reduction a P.O.P. is worn for 6–12 weeks; reduction or stabilisation with plates and screws may be necessary with double fractures that are often unstable.

Commonly in children a GREENSTICK fracture is produced which is easily reduced and heals in 4–6 weeks.

Powerful muscles act in the forearm to rotate the hand and move the wrist and fingers, and after a fracture the two segments of each bone may show variations in the degree of rotation that have to be corrected for perfect alignment and function.

FRACTURE-DISLOCATION of the lower radius and dislocation of the inferior radio-ulnar joint (Galeazzi fracture) is uncommon and usually needs an operation and fixation with P.O.P. for 12 weeks.

COLLES' FRACTURE . . . the commonest of all fractures, more often in the elderly, occurs with a fall on to the dorsi-flexed (bent-back) hand breaking the radius transversely just above the wrist and tilting it backwards, with some twisting towards the outer side. The classical dinner-fork deformity may be seen, and the pain, swelling and lack of movement at the wrist are noticeable.

Treatment: a Colles' plaster is worn for 6 weeks.

In a child the same fall produces a fracture-dislocation of the lower radial epiphysis (often called a SLIPPED EPIPHYSIS).

Treatment: as Colles.

With forward displacement of the lower fragment (palmar direction) the fracture is called a SMITH'S FRACTURE, and the P.O.P. is applied with the forearm supinated (Palm-up) for 6 weeks.

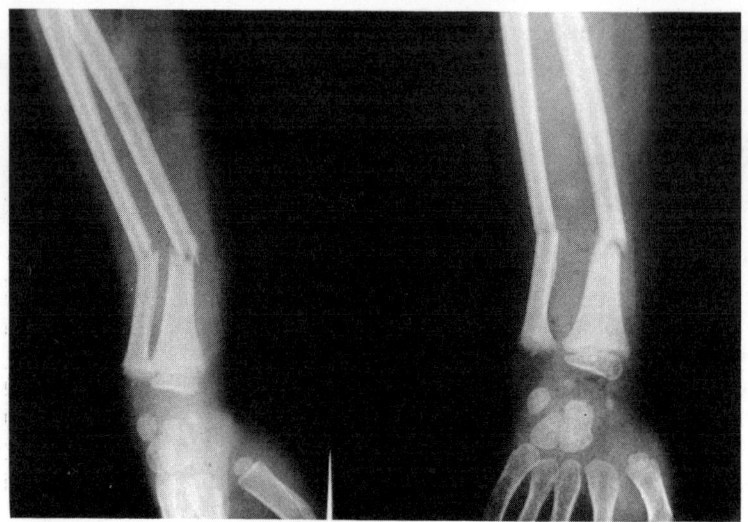

Xray showing fracture of both radius and ulna

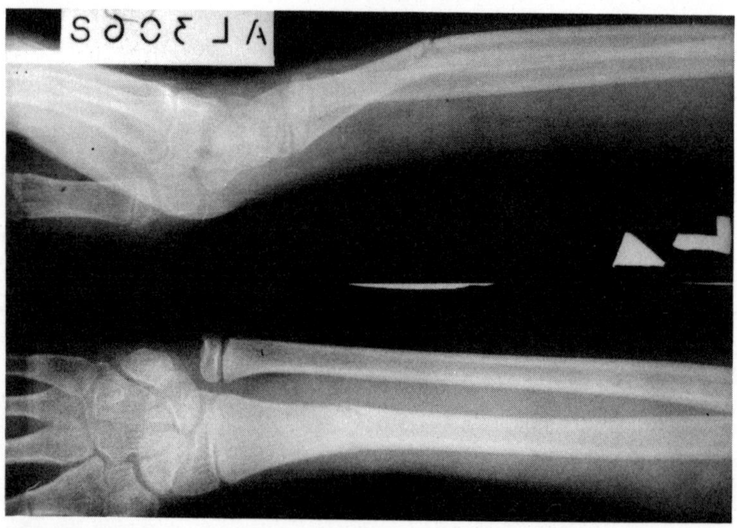

Xray of greenstick fracture of radius (bone ends not displaced)

TENOSYNOVITIS. . . due to overactivity in the flexor tendons at the wrist or on the dorsum of the hand, commonly due to playing repeated overhead smash at tennis which requires a rapid movement of the wrist tendons. Swelling within the tendon sheaths or tenderness on pressure with movement of the fingers and wrist are diagnostic.
Treatment: rest- strapping for 1–3 weeks (occasionally P.O.P.), heat and steroid injections.

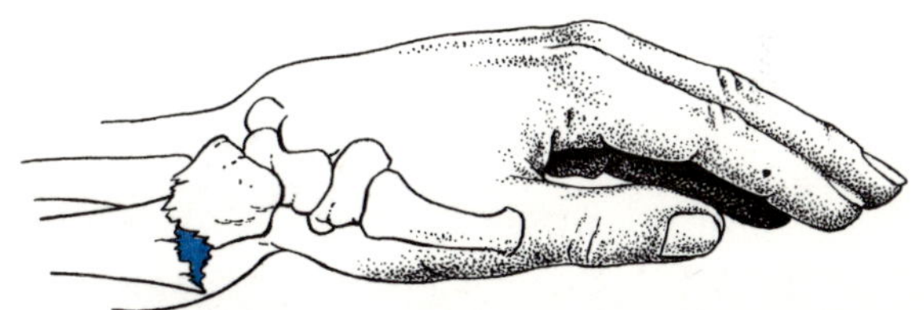

Colles fracture, showing the tilt of lower part of the radius

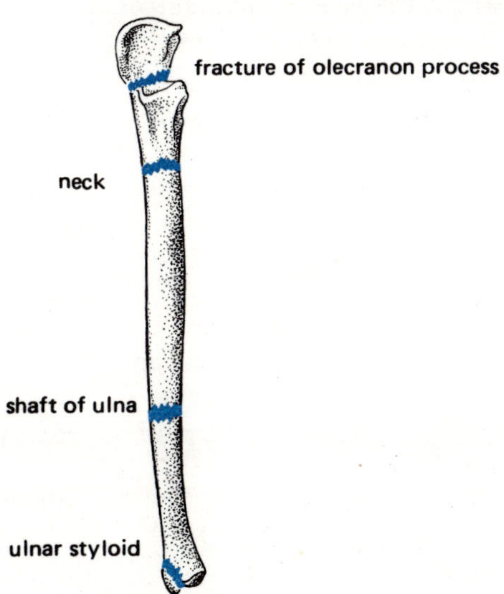

Fractures of ulna

Injuries to the Wrist and Hand

There are twenty-seven small bones in this region and any of the carpal, metacarpal or phalangeal bones may be fractured or dislocated.

FRACTURE OF THE SCAPHOID is the most important by far, since it is the main ball-bearing of the wrist around which movements take place. It is commonly fractured by a fall on to the dorsiflexed hand, and may fracture in three places. Tenderness is found in the anatomical snuff-box, with often very little swelling and pain. A FRACTURE MAY NOT SHOW ON X-RAY FOR THREE WEEKS and all suspected cases should be treated as a fracture with a scaphoid plaster during this period. The danger is avascular necrosis of the bone due to an interference with the blood supply of the proximal segment (adjacent to radius).

Treatment: P.O.P. for as long as the fracture is evident on X-ray, up to 12 weeks or so; however, prolonged immobilisation may lead to joint stiffness and the medical advisor may risk non-union after a certain period rather than prolong the plaster-immobilisation. Fractures of the waist (1) and proximal pole (2) may lead to avascular necrosis. Fractures of the tubercle (3) are of minor importance and can be treated with strapping or P.O.P. for a short duration.

SPRAINS OF THE WRIST ARE VERY RARE, ALWAYS EXCLUDE A FRACTURED SCAPHOID.

FRACTURE OF THE FIRST METACARPAL is usually sustained by a boxer when punching, but accompanies a difficult slip-catch at cricket. There is a localised swelling and tenderness at the base of the thumb.

Treatment: P.O.P. for 3–4 weeks, or strapping. Boxing can be resumed after 8–12 weeks.

BENNETT'S FRACTURE is a fracture of the base of the first metacarpal plus a dislocation from the trapezium bone resulting in instability. Thus operation and metallic fixation are often required, but a P.O.P. may suffice for 3–6 weeks.

FRACTURES OF THE METACARPALS AND PHALANGES . . . are common after minor trauma (usually cricket, boxing, goalkeeping, baseball and wrestling) and are treated with strapping or P.O.P. Sometimes internal operative fixation is needed. Fractures of the metacarpal necks produce a lump in the palm or an angulation on the back of the hand, reduction under an anaesthetic is carried out if the displacement interferes with normal function or appearance.

A MALLET FINGER (baseball finger) occurs when the terminal phalanx (tip of the finger) is knocked and the insertion of the extensor tendon torn. The tip falls forwards and only a small amount of movement is possible. It is common in rugger, wicket-keeping and goal-keeping.

Treatment: splintage for 3–6 weeks.

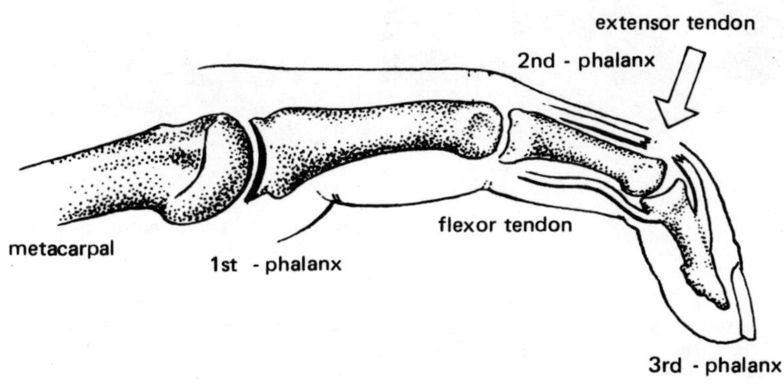

Illustration showing rupture of extensor tendon (mallet finger or baseball finger)

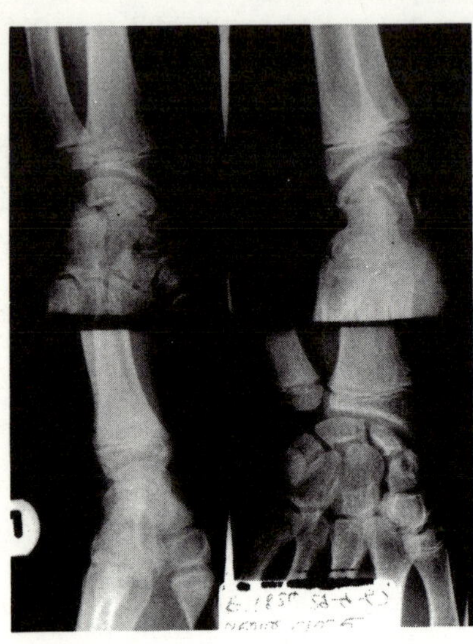

Xray showing fracture in scaphoid

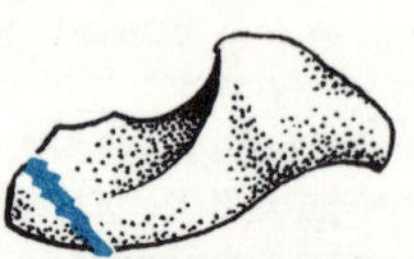

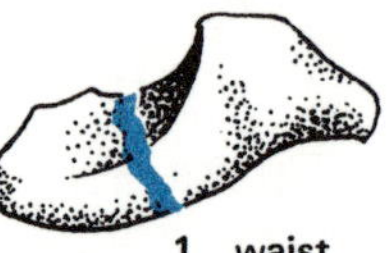

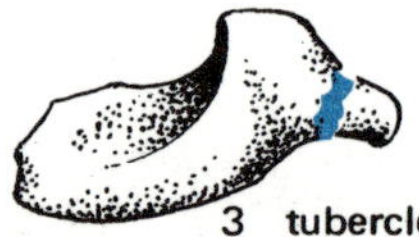

Illustration showing fracture of scaphoid

A special CHRONIC THICKENING is found just above the radial styloid with over-use of the thumb, it is called de Quervain's syndrome. Wringing movements of the wrist are painful, swelling and tenderness are found over the tendons concerned, with a palpable thickening and creaking sensation imparted to the examining fingers.

Treatment: a simple operation under local anaesthetic to divide the fibrous bands. Goalkeepers, gymnasts and volley-ball players are liable to both forms of tenosynovitis.

In **Rowing,** tenosynovitis of the wrist is commonly encountered especially in the early stages of training, and is due to a prolonged grip of the oar handle. Once it begins rowing aggravates the condition, and complete rest is essential until it subsides. Blisters are common on the fingers and palms. Muscular sprains are found in the shoulders, back and abdomen, usually early in the season or with faulty technique. Teaching the crews to keep a firm back at the beginning of a stroke can prevent lumbar disc disorders.

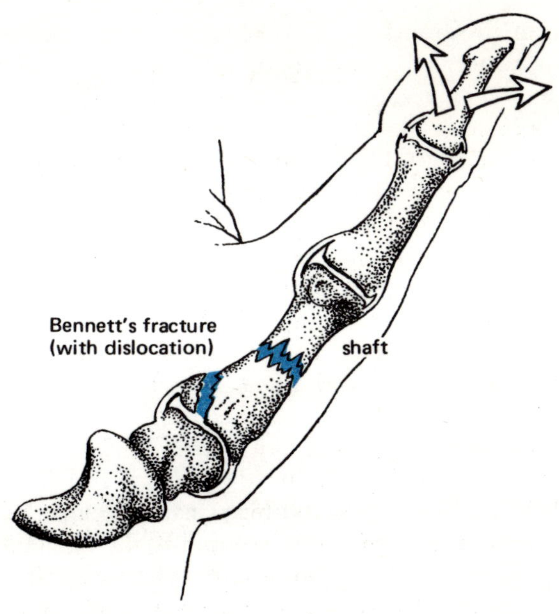

Illustration showing fracture of first metacarpal (thumb)

DISLOCATION OF THE FINGER may be found at the interphalangeal joints and can be reduced immediately by pulling the finger. A similar injury at the metacarpo-phalangeal joint may be more difficult to diagnose and be associated with a fracture.

Treatment: strapping for 1–3 weeks.

SPRAINS of the capsule, ligaments and soft tissues around the finger joints are very common especially in goalkeepers, volley-ball, water-polo etc. The swelling may persist for several months or indefinitely.

Treatment: strapping if severe for 1–3 weeks.

OSTEOARTHRITIS of the finger joints is found in cricketers, usually spinners who continually twist the finger-tips. The joints become swollen and deformed.

Treatment: heat, analgesics, physiotherapy.

Injuries to the Chest

Are often produced by a kick on the ribs (soccer, American football, rugger etc.) and boxing. There may be bruising of the soft tissue or a fracture of the ribs. During such injuries the sharp pointed ends of the ribs may be driven inwards and puncture the lung, liver or spleen. Damage to the lung results in a loss of the normal negative pressure within the pleural cavity which keeps the lungs firmly applied to the inner aspect of the chest wall, so that the lung loses this connection and does not passively follow the movement of the chest, i.e. inspiration does not occur in that lung. THIS CONDITION IS VERY SERIOUS. The player complains of the initial pain of the fractured rib(s), followed by a shortness of breath, with an occasional thumping sensation from the heart which is either displaced slightly or not surrounded by the lung tissue on one side. Such injuries need URGENT TRANSFER TO HOSPITAL. Blows over the heart usually cause no trouble.

Puncture wounds from a sharp point, i.e. javelin, allow air to escape from the chest and usually collapse the lung. The hole should be covered with a sterile dressing and the athlete taken to hospital.

FRACTURED RIBS do NOT need strapping, for this treatment may press the sharp ends internally, or if strapped too tightly it stops the normal respiratory excursion of the lung tissue so that stagnation and infection supervene.

Treatment: analgesics or an injection of a long-acting local anaesthetic.

MULTIPLE rib fractures require hospitalisation and stabilisation with pins or wires (flail chest syndrome).

RIB STRESS FRACTURES are found after overuse of the chest muscles as in tennis, and rowing. Respond to rest.

TEARS OF THE PECTORALIS MAJOR (and rarely MINOR) occurs with excessive pushing or lifting (as in weight-lifting or gymnastics). Pain and tenderness is found over the insertion of this muscle on the ribs close to the sternum. Treatment: rest, heat, analgesics.

Tenderness over the costal cartilages is sometimes complained of by a player; usually it is a variety of costo-chondritis (Tietz syndrome) and heals spontaneously. Treatment: as tears.

N.B. Disorders of the thoracic spine cause a radiation of pain around the chest wall and can stimulate chest conditions.

Cricketers are prone to fractured ribs when hit by a 5½ oz. ball travelling at 80–90 miles per hour. Blows on the fingers are also common despite the use of batting gloves, and wrist and forearm fractures are seen. The legs, largely protected by pads when batting, are seldom seriously injured but the feet are often hit by a full pitched ball which may result in severe bruising or even a fracture. Blows on the scrotum cause a haematoma, and protection can be afforded by an aluminium protector. Slipping on a wet-wicket can cause a ruptured Achilles tendon or pulled hamstring. Sudden twisting when bending at fielding may cause lumbar strain or a slipped disc. Ligamentous and meniscal damage may be produced in the knee.

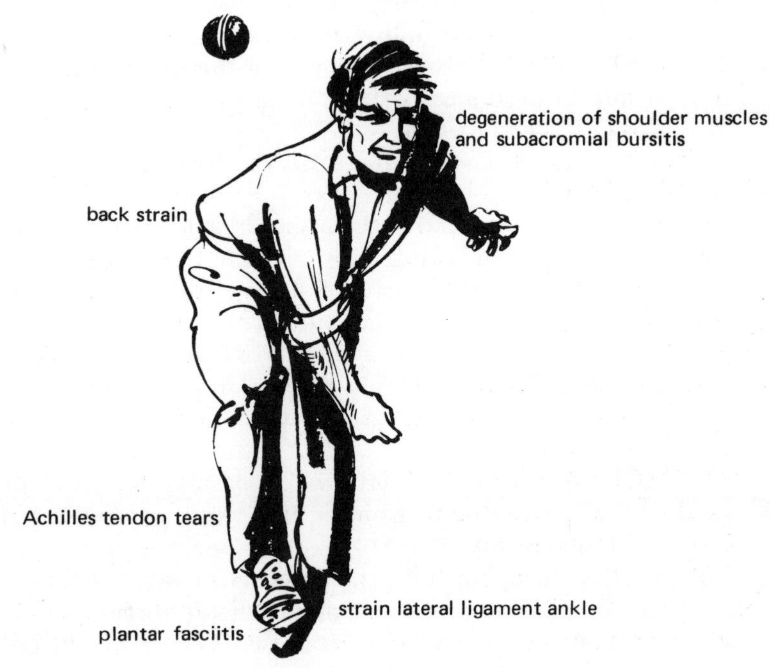

Injuries to the Abdomen

Direct blows onto the abdomen rarely injure the contents because of the protection of the strong abdominal muscles and the mobility of many of the contained organs. Relatively fixed structures are the most frequently damaged leading to bleeding which may vary from a small bruise to several litres.

THE SYMPTOMS AND SIGNS OF AN INTRA-ABDOMINAL INJURY ARE:

1. PAIN may be localised over the injured area or referred to the centre of the abdomen. With diaphragmatic irritation, from blood, intestinal contents etc. the pain is felt over the tip of the shoulder.
2. SHOCK due to bleeding, characterised by a rapid pulse, sweating, anxiety, cold pale extremities.
3. RIGID ABDOMEN from spasm of the muscles of the abdomen due to peritoneal irritation.
4. VOMITING or nausea.
5. The passage of blood in the urine or motions.

LIVER INJURY follows a severe blow over the right lower ribs. Shock may be rapid and R. shoulder tip pain evident.

SPLEEN . . . injured with a blow over the L. lower ribs. Shock often rapid, but may be delayed for up to 3 weeks (delayed rupture). L. shoulder-tip pain evident.

KIDNEY . . . injured with a blow over either loin. Bleeding may be concealed or suddenly appear in the urine. May be microscopic or obvious. All specimens should be examined for twenty-four hours.

TESTICULAR INJURY follows a scrotal blow and often produces a haematoma which may need aspiration in a Casualty Department.

URETHRA. Bleeding from the external meatus on the tip of the penis is VERY serious and may indicate disruption of the urethra. May be associated with a FRACTURED PELVIS. URGENT HOSPITALISATION. The player MUST NOT

PASS URINE, or attempt to.

The above injuries are SERIOUS and to avoid shock transport the athlete quickly but gently.

HAEMATOMAS & SPRAINS of the abdominal muscles are of minor importance and rapidly heal with rest. Hernias in athletes need surgical correction to prevent nipping during exercise, full activity is accomplished after a 9–12 week lay-off following operation.

N.B. Thoracic (lower) and Lumbar spine disorders can cause radiation of pain around the abdomen and simulate abdominal conditions.

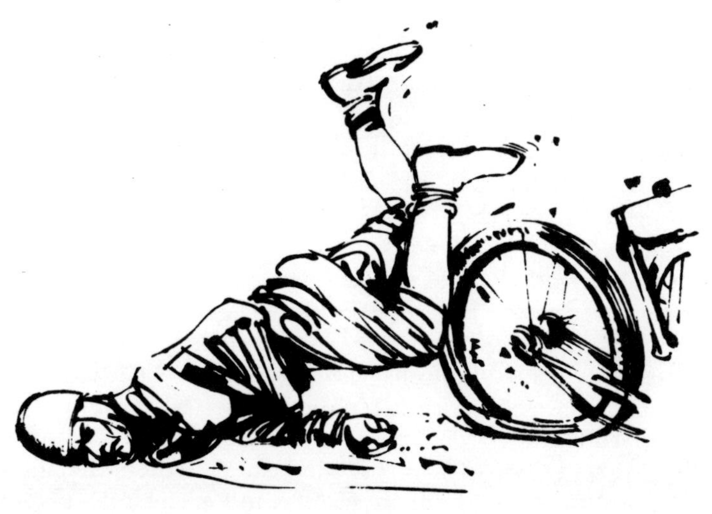

Damage to shoulder and cervical spine
Nerve roots (brachial plexus) to the arm may be stretched and torn

Injuries to the Hip and Pelvis

FRACTURES OF THE PELVIS. These are uncommon in sport except after riding injuries when the horse rolls over the rider's pelvis. Either of the three bones (ilium, pubis, or ischium) can be damaged, but a fracture in one or more pubic rami is by far the most common. Bruising and tenderness is evident over the pelvis, with a varying degree of pain. The patient may be able to walk but with some difficulty. DAMAGE to the bladder, bowel and urethra may co-exist.

Treatment: Bed rest for 3–6 weeks.

TENDERNESS OVER THE LOWER BUTTOCK, confined to the ischial bones, may result from chronic avulsion of small flakes of bone from the pull of the hamstrings as in hurdling.

FRACTURES OF THE FEMORAL NECK are very uncommon in athletes except cyclists, but usually found in the elderly after a fall. The diagnosis rests on the presence of shortening of the leg with external rotation of the foot.

Treatment: bed rest and traction, or pinning operation. No weight-bearing for 3 months.

STRESS FRACTURES are rarely seen in the femoral neck, and heal with rest (see Tibia).

SLIPPED EPIPHYSIS. Here the fracture extends through the epiphyseal cartilage. It may occur suddenly after a blow, or gradually over several weeks. ALWAYS found in the 10–15 years old period. Pain is complained of in the hip, but sometimes referred to the KNEE. It is often regarded as a sprain and ignored. Limping becomes more pronounced as the condition progresses. Such symptoms should always AROUSE SUSPICION in a school child; children do NOT limp for no reason. (In the 5–10 year group the same picture is found with PERTHES' DISEASE or pseudocoxalgia when the femoral head loses some of its blood supply and necroses). This condition also warrants urgent treatment by traction, bed rest and weight-relieving calipers or slings for up to 2 years, as in slipped epiphysis.

DISLOCATION OF THE HIP may be anterior or posterior (more common, when the sciatic nerve is liable to damage). The hip joint is very strong and excessive force is needed to inflict such an injury (motor accidents). Great pain and limitation of movement is found in the region of the hip.

Treatment: reduction under G.A.

SUBTROCHANTERIC FRACTURES occur in the upper shaft of the femur, may require traction, P.O.P. or internal fixation. Rare in athletes.

In SWIMMING injuries are uncommon. In the front and back crawl the leg action is a powerful up-and-down movement by repeated flexion and extension at the hip. Tears may be occasionally found in the quadriceps. In the breast stroke a vigorous adduction of both legs is needed and tears of the adductor longus are found. Minor tears of the medial and coronary ligaments (with cartilage trouble) are seen in the knee. Many of the small shoulder muscles become painful after prolonged use, especially in the front crawl when the hand is lifted repeatedly from the water and carried forward with a rotational action.

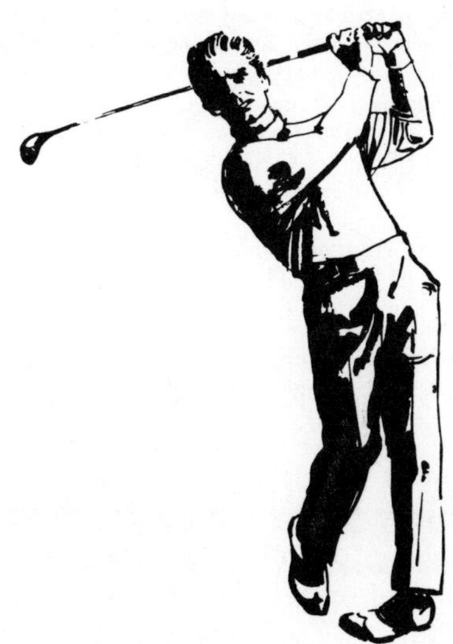

Golfers are prone to sprains of the cervical and lumbar spines, shoulder and knee.

Injuries to the Thigh

FRACTURES OF THE FEMUR SHAFT. These are very serious injuries since at least two pints (1L) of blood are lost into the thigh muscles, and the patient becomes shocked. Direct force, either a kick or a blow, produces a transverse fracture, while a spiral fracture is caused by a fall in which the foot is anchored and a twisting force is applied to the body, usually from a collision with another player. The sickening crack, severe pain, swelling of the thigh and shocked condition are diagnostic.

Treatment: Immediate splinting and removal of the player on a stretcher. In hospital a transfusion is given and the leg subjected to rest and traction for 12 weeks. A Kuntscher nail is used for upper third fractures—the nail being hammered down the shaft of the femur to stabilise the fracture.

SUPRACONDYLAR FRACTURES are rare and confined to adults. The femur is fractured above the condyles with the lower segment tilted backwards by the pull of the gastrocnemius. The knee is very swollen and painful with a tender area above the patella (or alongside).

Treatment: 12 weeks traction or pinning with nails or screws.

FRACTURES OF THE FEMORAL CONDYLES are due to a direct fall on the leg driving the tibia against the condyles. In adolescence and childhood the femoral epiphysis can separate.

Diagnosis and treatment: as for supracondylar.

RECURRENT GROIN INJURY. This condition is produced by rapid acceleration forces in soccer, sprinting, hurdling, long-jumping etc. which partially or completely tears the insertion of the ADDUCTOR LONGUS TENDON at its origin from the pubic bone. An early return to activity will result in a recurrence; at least four weeks of complete rest are needed. When this injury occurs the athlete suddenly stops in his tracks and limps to the touchline complaining of pain in the groin. Tenderness is found over the insertion, with weakness or pain on attempting adduction against resistance. (Breast stroke swimming, with its unusual leg action, often produces chronic adductor tendinitis, so do repeated sliding tackles at soccer).

Treatment: rest, static, passive and active exercises as graduated physiotherapy over several weeks, with heat, analgesics and ultrasound. Manipulation under anaesthetic has been advocated in chronic cases.

CALCIFICATION IN THE ADDUCTOR LONGUS TENDON is seen in horse riders who repeatedly grip the horses flanks with the thighs. Recurrent inflammation (PERITENDINITIS) can occur around the tendon without calcification.

Treatment: as above.

TEARS OF THE ILIO-PSOAS, RECTUS FEMORIS, SARTORIUS are occasionally found. Tenderness is detected over their points of origin or insertion.

Treatment: as above.

FRACTURES OF THE FEMUR

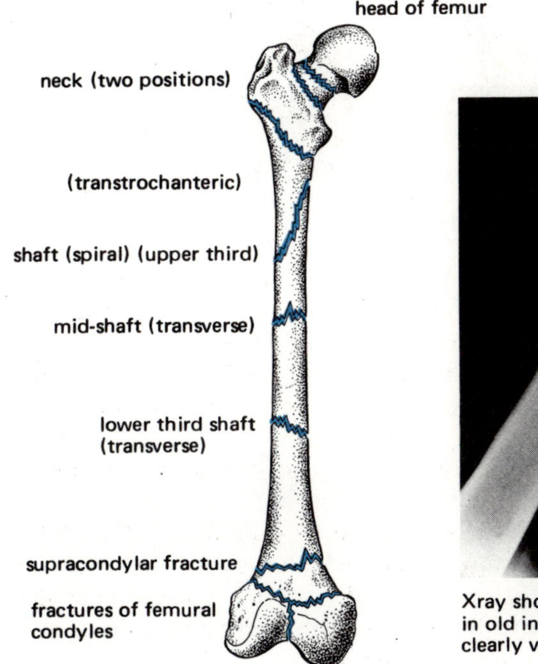

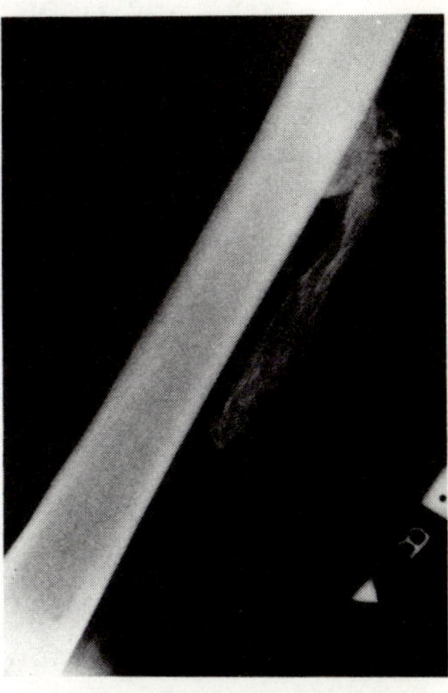

Xray showing myositis ossificans in old injury of thigh. New bone clearly visible connected to femur

MUSCLES OF THIGH

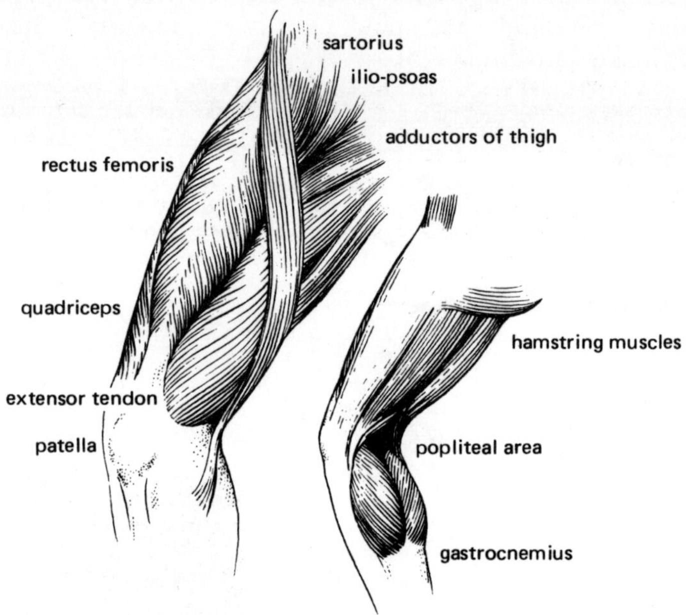

PULLED HAMSTRINGS ARE also common in sprinting activities and produce weakness in the follow-through action of the unsupported leg during running. Tearing can occur at several points (see muscle injury). Pain is felt when the hamstrings are stretched, typically when sitting down, and may radiate down the leg.

Treatment: rest, heat, physiotherapy as for muscle injuries. (p.18)

Tenderness over the greater trochanter (TROCHANTERIC BURSITIS) is found after repeated abduction and rotation of the hip (batsmen in cricket) and pain is produced over the outer side of the hip, radiating down the leg or into the groin.

Treatment: rest, heat and analgesics.

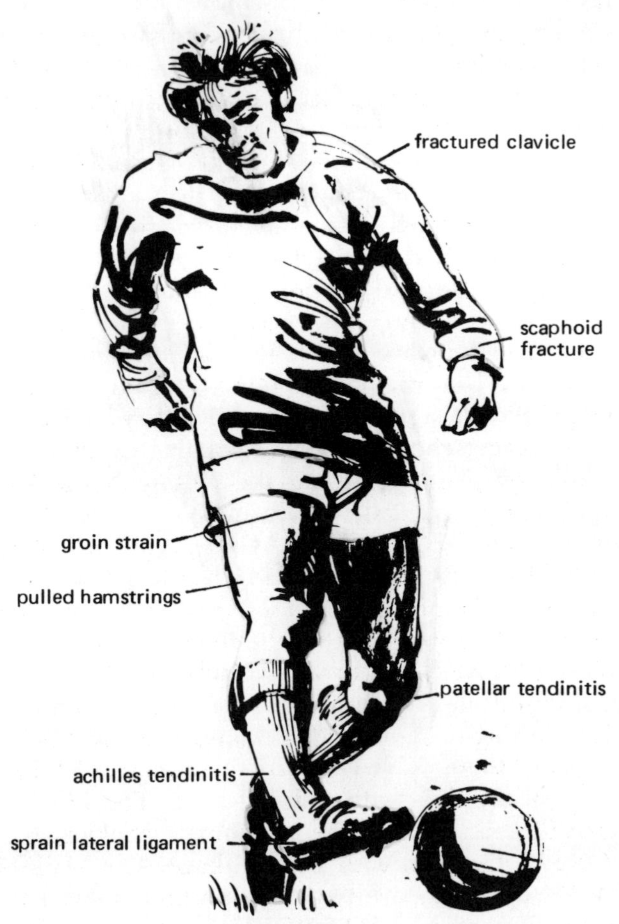
fractured clavicle
scaphoid
fracture
groin strain
pulled hamstrings
patellar tendinitis
achilles tendinitis
sprain lateral ligament

Injuries to the Knee

Are classed as a) bony, b) ligamentous and c) cartilaginous. When examining the knee, always compare the other side. (This also applies to the examination of all limb injuries). Pain in the knee may be referred from the hip. The five common symptoms of knee trouble are pain, swelling, stiffness, limp and mechanical trouble (locking, instability, clicking). Test the full range of movement and detect abnormal mobility with the knee extended. Normally there should be no movement with an extended knee. Observe the patella, its shape and whether it can be tapped against the femoral condyles (it does not articulate with the tibia) indicating an effusion, which spreads for 3 to 4 inches above the joint beneath the anterior thigh muscles (suprapatellar bursa). Pain produced by tapping the patella against the condyles may indicate hyaline cartilage damage (chondromalacia patellae). Observe rotation of the tibia by gently grasping the foot with the knee fully flexed and gently turning the foot in and out. In McMURRAY'S test for INTERNAL CARTILAGE DAMAGE the foot is EXTERNALLY ROTATED and the flexed knee straightened, and as the bony surfaces pass over the torn cartilage a click may be heard or a jump felt by the fingers resting on the joint line. With EXTERNAL cartilage trouble the leg is gently extended from full flexion with INTERNAL rotation of the foot and the same signs found. With damage to the ANTERIOR CRUCIATE there is an abnormal forward (ANTERIOR) movement of the tibia with a flexed knee. The POSTERIOR CRUCIATE is tested by pushing backwards (POSTERIORLY) the tibia with a flexed knee. The MEDIAL and LATERAL ligaments are tested by pushing against the inner or outer aspect of an EXTENDED knee while grasping the leg with the other hand. Weakness is indicated by a rocking movement. Very slight degrees of mobility are found with effusions.

Treatment: rest, elevation, compression, bed rest and traction for effusion if severe, with surgery for ligamentous tears and cartilage damage. Active and passive movements, static exercises etc. THE KEY TO SUCCESSFUL RECOVERY OF A KNEE INJURY RESIDES IN STRONG AND HEALTHY QUADRICEPS. No knee will recover good function unless the quadriceps are powerful. The most important member is the Vastus medialis, prominent on the lower inner aspect of the thigh, and INSERTED DIRECTLY INTO THE PATELLA. After knee injuries the quadriceps begins to atrophy within 2–3 days, especially the Vastus medialis, and these muscles should be assessed regularly. If any atrophy is detected isometric (static) exercises should be encouraged. Before athletic exercise is undertaken the quadriceps must be strengthened by weight-bearing exercise.

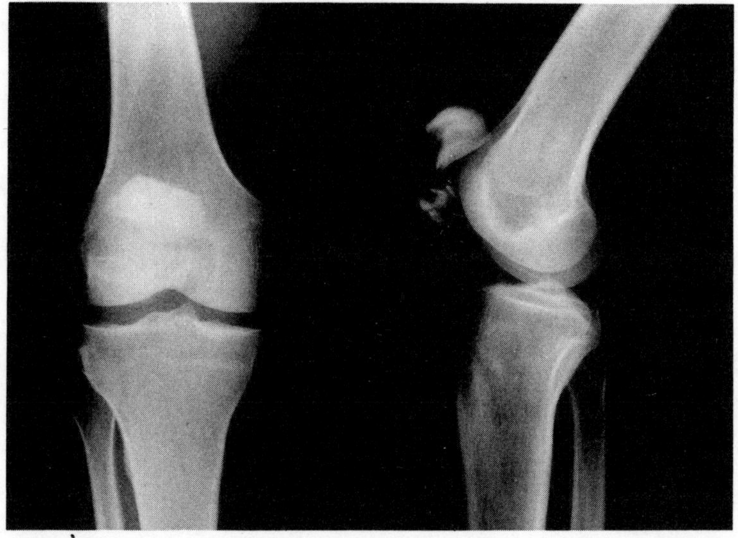

Xray showing transverse fracture of patella

TRAUMATIC EFFUSION may be synovial, blood or both. With a significant amount of blood in the joint a 'doughy' feeling can be palpated. All blood should be aspirated in Casualty Department to prevent adhesions (see joints). As the swelling subsides with rest etc. active and passive movements are carried out. The quadriceps should be maintained by static exercises.

FRACTURE OF THE TIBIAL CONDYLES and tibial spine occur with direct trauma or a fall on a bending knee. In the latter case the cruciate ligaments take all the force and if they do not tear their insertion into the tibial spines may become detached as a bony flake. The diagnosis is by pain, sudden swelling (boggy) and inability to move the knee.

Treatment: rest and P.O.P. for 6–12 weeks. Operation and elevation of the tibial condyles to produce a smooth articular surface for the femur, with metallic fixation, may be necessary,

FRACTURES OF THE PATELLA are often due to direct violence (kick on the knee or fall), but can follow a powerful quadriceps contraction with the foot stationary, so that the full force of the tendon is exerted on the bone. The knee rapidly becomes swollen and painful, and a palpable gap in the subcutaneous surface of the patella is obvious.

Treatment: suturing or metallic fixation with P.O.P. immobilisation for 6–12 weeks, followed by gentle physiotherapy and stretching of the tendon. If the patella is badly damaged (comminuted) it is better to excise the bone, for any irregularity in its surface wears the hyaline cartilage of the femoral condyles.

STRESS FRACTURES are sometimes observed in the patella. They heal with rest and P.O.P. for 4 weeks (see Tibia).

DISLOCATION OF THE PATELLA is invariably in a lateral direction and can be seen. It is easily reduced but may become recurrent when an operation is needed.

DISLOCATION OF THE KNEE is caused by severe violence e.g. diving tackle at rugger, riding injury; usually the knee is extended and the leg driven backwards by the deforming forces. It is a serious injury since the ligaments and cartilages are torn, and the vessels and nerves on the back of the knee may be damaged. Thus the pulse and sensation must be tested in the limb concerned. The diagnosis is made from the gross pain and deformity.

Treatment: reduction, operative treatment, with P.O.P. for 12 weeks.

CHONDROMALACIA PATELLAE is found in cyclists, or in other sports with repeated minor falls on the knee. The hyaline cartilage on the posterior surface of the patella becomes roughened and reddened. The person complains of pain on going upstairs and of occasional swelling. Later the knee tends to give way but true locking does not occur. Pressing the patella against the femoral condyles

produces pain. Squatting or sitting with the knee bent aggravates the pain.
Treatment: rest and physiotherapy. In severe cases the patella can be excised.
OSTEOCHONDRITIS DISSECANS occurs when a tiny segment of bone in the knee joint becomes ischaemic from repeated minor trauma, usually on the medial femoral condyle. It gives rise to pain, loose body locking, and instability. An X-ray shows the lesion.
Treatment: an operation is required to drill and fix, or excise, the affected segment.
Occasionally a BIPARTITE PATELLA (consisting of two bones instead of one) is found. Usually they cause no symptoms, rarely the smaller fragment may become partially detached and cause pain and tenderness.
Treatment: rest, crepe 2–4 weeks.
Injections of steroids into the knee joint may give rise to cartilage damage resembling osteochondritis (see steroid injections).
HOCKEY PLAYERS seldom collide and most injuries are due to the ball and stick. Blows on the knees produce an effusion, but on rough grounds the ball can fly in any direction and cuts and abrasions are common, especially on the face. Shin-guards can protect against leg injuries. Sudden turning and stopping can produce knee and hip troubles. Collision with an opponent's goalkeeper may cause broken ribs, concussion etc.

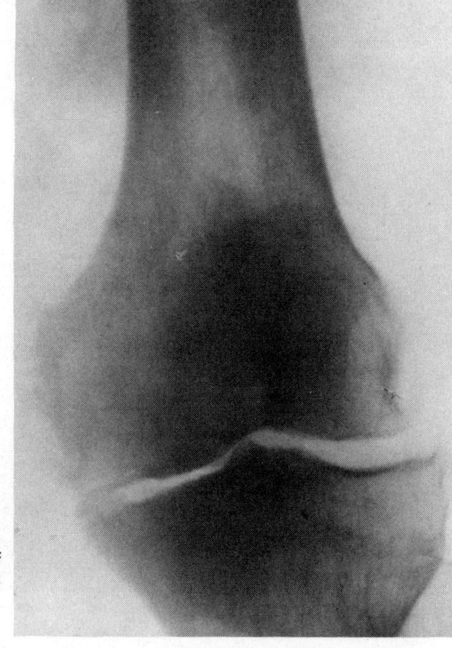

Xray showing osteoarthritis of knee (blurring of normal bone contour, irregularity of joint space)

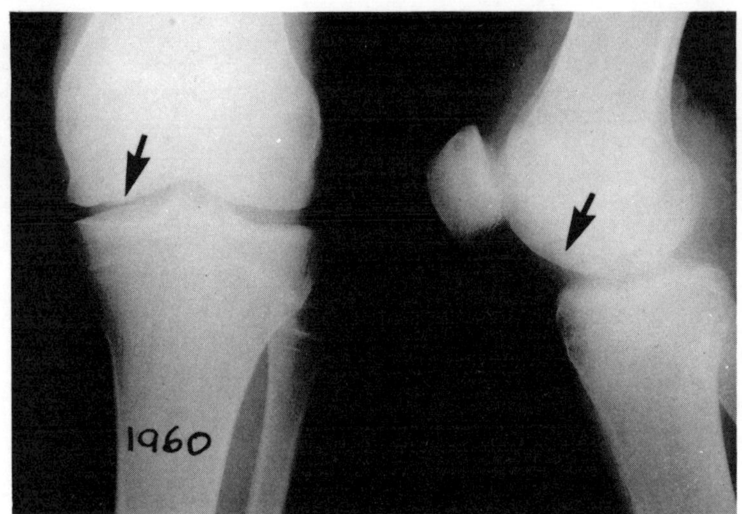

Xray showing osteochondritis dissecans (small piece of bone loose)

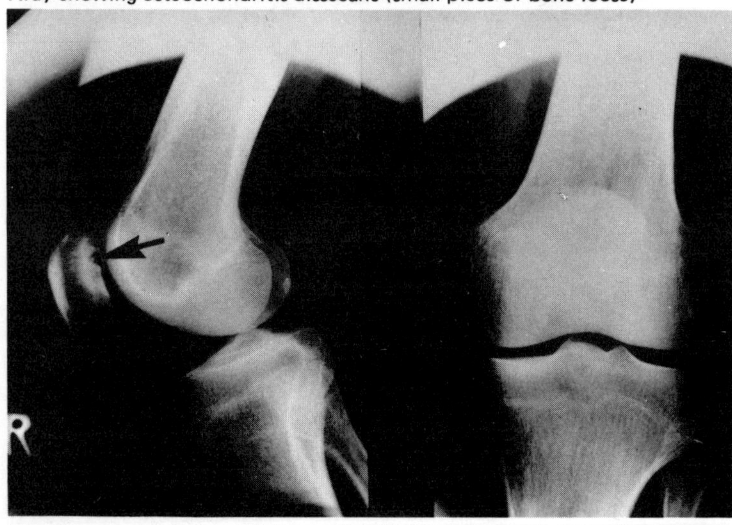

Xray showing chondromalacia patellae (softening of articular surface shown by rough surface)

Injuries to the Knees

LIGAMENTS. Each ligament may be injured on its own or with others, producing a bewildering number of ligamentous injuries. Most torn ligaments should be repaired surgically shortly after injury since, once the knee becomes unstable, it is subjected to repeated trauma and atrophy of the thigh muscles follows. Later other compensatory ligaments may weaken and ultimately osteoarthritis supervenes.

Damage to the ligaments may co-exist with bony and meniscal injury. The most frequent mechanisms by which the ligaments of the knee are injured are:

(a) HYPEREXTENSION—This motion ruptures the
- (i) anterior cruciate
- (ii) stretches the capsule posteriorly
- (iii) posterior cruciate (partially)

(b) ANTERIOR OR POSTERIOR DISPLACEMENT OF TIBIA ON THE FEMUR WITH FLEXED KNEE.
- (i) anterior cruciate damaged with excessive anterior movement.
- (ii) posterior cruciate damaged with excessive posterior movement.

(c) VALGUS (LATERAL MOVEMENT OF FOOT) MOTION, FLEXION AND INTERNAL ROTATION OF FEMUR ON TIBIA. (sudden turn inwards).
- (i) tears superficial layers of tibial (medial) ligament.
- (ii) then deep layers of tibial (medial) ligament.
- (iii) ruptures anterior cruciate ligament (caused by rotation.
- (iv) tears the medial meniscus.
- (v) causes flake fracture of the anterior tibial spine.
- (vi) causes fracture of the lateral tibial condyle.

(d) VARUS (MEDIAL MOVEMENT OF FOOT), FLEXION AND EXTERNAL ROTATION OF THE FEMUR ON TIBIA. (sudden turn outwards).

(i) injury to fibular (lateral) ligament.
(ii) tears anterior cruciate.
(iii) tears fibres of popliteus.
(iv) fractures medial tibial condyle.
(v) tears lateral meniscus

The functions of the ligaments of the knee are so interrelated and injuries to a single ligament so uncommon, that all cases of 'sprained knees' or 'effusions' should be examined for ligamentous instability (see knee injuries).

Haematoma, pain, swelling, tenderness, excessive movement and instability are the main complaints. Valgus rocking of the tibia on the femur with the knee extended suggests rupture of both medial (tibial) collateral and anterior cruciate (which also gives anterior instability). Valgus rocking with the knee very slightly flexed but absent when the knee is extended indicates rupture of the medial ligament alone, this injury is commonly missed for the swelling gravitates to the calf, and the player walks by bracing the quadriceps. In the case of single ligament damage X-rays may be necessary to detect the degree of movement permitted between the tibia and femur, thus separating partial collateral ligament damage from total rupture. The most vital and vulnerable structure of the knee is the medial ligament, commonly injured in American football, soccer with a hard tackle from the outer aspect, in a scrum collapse at rugger, or when an opponent falls against the outer side of an extended leg.

Treatment: for partial tears, rest in plaster for 3–6 weeks; for the complete tears, surgical sutures and P.O.P. for 6 weeks.

Injury to the anterior cruciate occurs when a player falls from mid-air (basketball, heading at soccer) with his leg doubled-up beneath him.

The anterior cruciate is injured much less commonly than the posterior and can be left without suturing—the quadriceps will compensate. Tenderness and swelling in the popliteal space indicates a haematoma from posterior capsule or posterior cruciate damage and may co-exist with anterior cruciate tears, later bruising appears in the calf. The posterior cruciate injury cannot be compensated for by the quadriceps and surgical intervention and sutures are required. This treatment is often unsuccessful (P.O.P. for 6 weeks). Flake fractures of the tibial spines with cruciate tears may need internal fixation if grossly detached. O'Donoghue described a severe athletic injury when the medial ligament, anterior cruciate and medial meniscus are injured in combination (The Unhappy Trial of O'Donoghue).

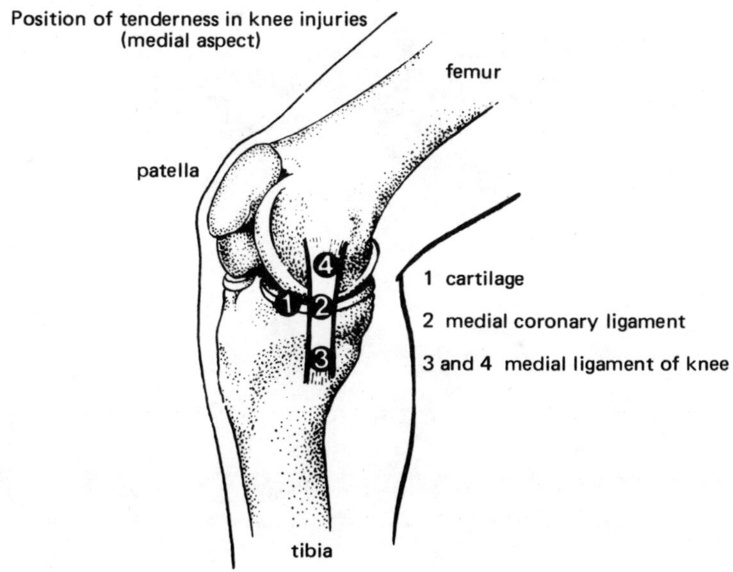

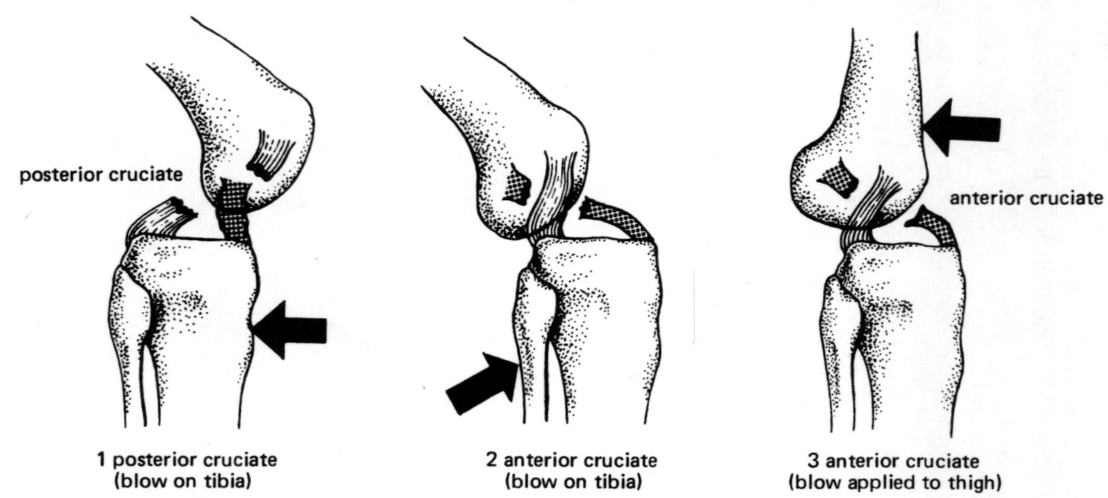

Illustration showing damage to ligaments within knee (normally ligaments from an X)

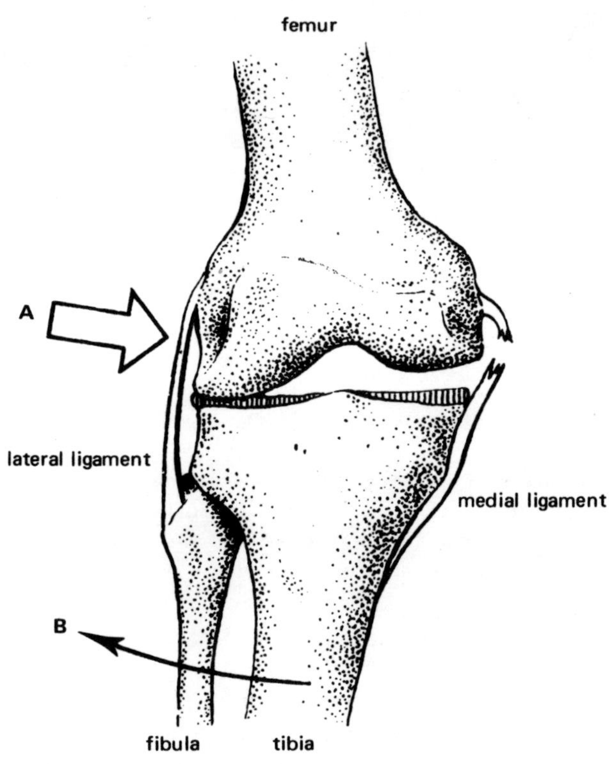

Illustration to show damage to the medial ligament (sprain or rupture) with a blow from either outer aspect knee (A) or inner aspect of ankle and foot (B).

Treatment for all knee injuries: rest, aspiration, compression, surgical suture, P.O.P. cylinder, changed at 3 weeks to allow gentle weight bearing, removed at 6 weeks; physiotherapy and quadriceps strengthening exercises.

Ski-ing accidents rarely damage the menisci, but the rotational forces usually partially tears the upper part of the medial ligament, which heals with rest etc.

Injuries to the Knees

MENISCAL DAMAGE. The two menisci (often called 'cartilages' since they consist of fibro-cartilage) are commonly injured during sports activities and require surgical excision. Once cartilaginous damage is diagnosed, removal is the correct treatment for ligamentous weakness and later osteoarthritis may develop.

Tears occur:—

(a) longitudinal or classic bucket-handle tears of the body.
(b) transverse tears of the body.
(c) oblique tears of the body.
(d) posterior horn tears.
(e) anterior horn tears.
(f) peripheral tears from the capsule, coronary ligaments etc.

A meniscus is torn by a rotating force carried out when the joint is partially flexed. This rotating force 'sucks' the meniscus concerned towards the centre of the joint when it is crushed between the extending tibia and femur.

Normally the shape, elasticity and peripheral attachments (medial ligament and medial coronary ligament for internal; popliteus muscle and lateral coronary ligament for external meniscus) keep them from moving centrally. Tears of the peripheral attachments by excessive rotational weight-bearing forces allow the menisci to be later forced towards the centre of the joint and damaged—classically a bucket-handle tear is produced. If a portion of cartilage becomes caught in the inter-condylar notch then locking follows.

N.B. Vigorous internal (medial) rotation of the femur on the tibia with the knee flexed and weight bearing traps an excessively mobile medial meniscus, and extension tears it.

Vigorous external (lateral) rotation of the femur on the tibia with the knee flexed and weight bearing traps an excessively mobile lateral meniscus, and extension tears it. (The lateral meniscus is not attached to the lateral fibular ligament, but to the popliteus muscle which pulls it out of harm's way, and to two small internal ligaments which cause it to follow the movements of the femur closely. Thus it is less frequently damaged than the medial).

The diagnosis—several minor knee troubles ultimately give rise to locking when the knee cannot be fully extended. Sometimes an effusion with snapping or clicking may be the sole complaint. A sensation of giving way in the knee, especially on rotary movements (usually posterior horn tears) or on going upstairs (quadriceps weakness) is found. Tenderness around the joint line may be detected (exclude collateral ligament and coronary ligament tears) and McMurray's test is often positive. Treatment: for the first locking episode—rest, traction and physiotherapy for 2–6 weeks. The displaced segment of a torn meniscus may be reduced manually as a palliative measure. The knee is flexed and the tibia grasped at the ankle. For a medial meniscus push the knee from the lateral side (valgus) to open out the medial joint space and rotate the foot medially. (For a lateral meniscus, rotate foot laterally with varus at knee i.e. pressure from inner aspect to open out lateral space). Recurrent damage needs surgical excision since tears of the body never heal, only small tears of the periphery; postoperative rest for 10 days with static exercises, then physiotherapy and full return to sports activity in 6–12 weeks.

CYSTS OF THE CARTILAGE. These present as a hard swelling (almost always laterally, at the level of the joint line). Due to repeated trauma to the meniscus, more prominent in extension. Usually needs surgical excision.

SNAPPING KNEE may be due to cysts of the menisci, discoid meniscus or tendons, especially popliteus.

DISCOID MENISCUS invariably on lateral aspect, usually cause no symptoms unless injured. The meniscus is 'disc-shaped' rather than the characteristic 'moon' shape.

TIBIAL (MEDIAL) COLLATERAL LIGAMENT SYNDROME present with tenderness over the medial aspect of joint, often aggravated by activity. The underlying trouble is a deformity of the medial meniscus from repeated minor injuries, leading to abnormal stretching of the medial ligament by the slightly displaced meniscus.

Treatment: meniscectomy.

RUGGER injuries are common, the knee and quadriceps injuries are produced by too sharp a turn especially when the ground is waterlogged so that the boots are inclined to stick while the legs move on. In a heavy tackle with the opponent falling across an extended knee, ligamentous damage is produced. A scrum collapse may also injure the shoulder and neck as well as the knee. Dislocated bones, especially fingers, are common when one person tries to handle the ball as another kicks on. An opponent may fall across a dribbling player's foot thus trapping it and fracturing the ankle or tibia. A player may be winded while making a 'mark' from a violent collision.

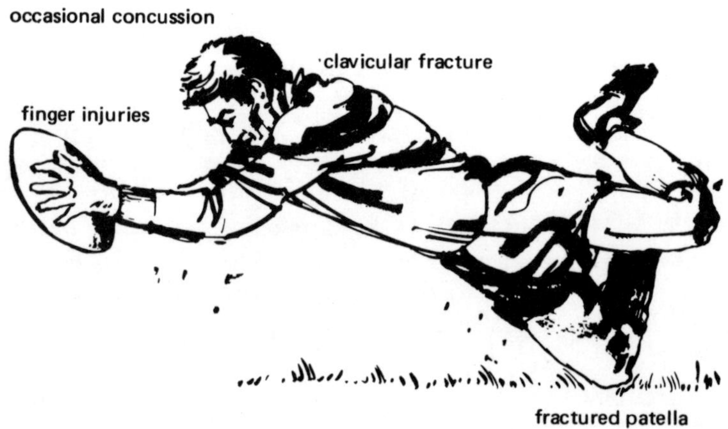

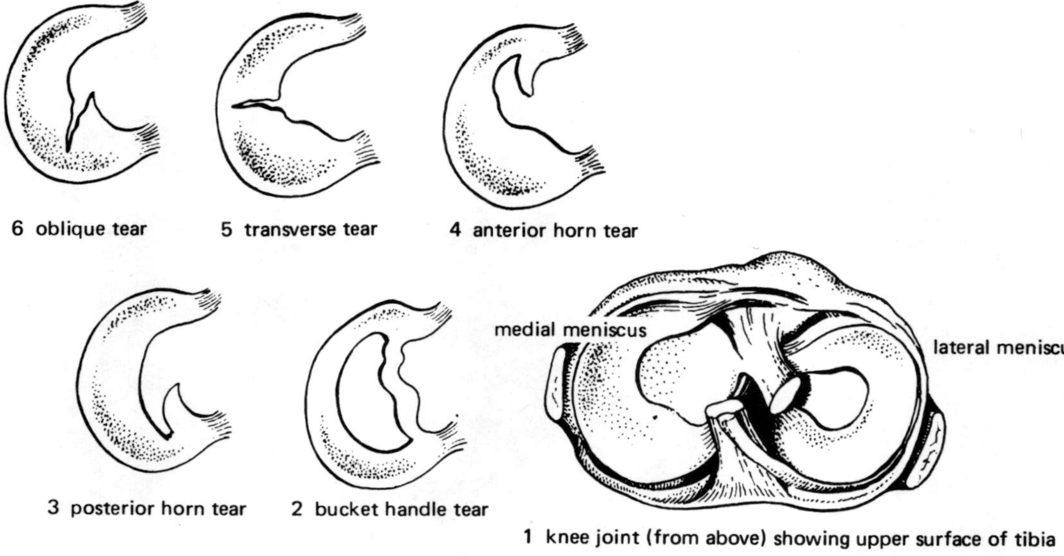

Illustration to show types of cartilage (meniscal) damage within knee

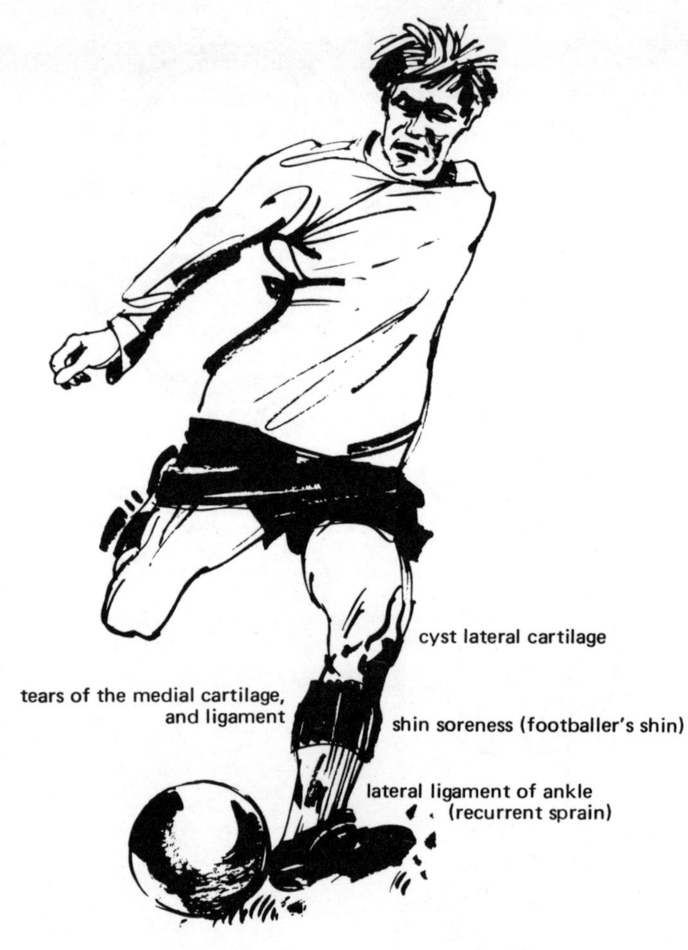

Twisting force to inner aspect of knee tears cartilages as the knee straightens

Other Knee Lesions

OSTEOARTHRITIS is uncommon in sportsmen except when the knee has been subjected to repeated injury, or ligamentous or cartilagenous damage has been ignored. The hyaline articular cartilage becomes rough, fibrillated and thinned, then pieces flake off. The bone beneath it scleroses and forms cysts. At the non-pressure areas the cartilage proliferates and calcifies, forming osteophytes which occasionally break off as loose bodies. Excess synovial fluid is produced by the synovial membrane, which proliferates. Diagnosis is apparent from the dull ache, worse after use, and it often hurts the sufferer to get going after sitting for any length of time. Swelling and bogginess may be detected. X-ray shows the characteristic appearance.

LOOSE BODIES cause locking and instability in the knee.

produced by a. injury and separation of a piece of bone or cartilage within the joint.

b. osteochondritis dissecans.

c. osteoarthritis.

d. fibrinous loose bodies from inflammation.

e. torn cartilage (meniscus).

f. small calcified, fatty or synovial nodules (osteochondromatosis).

A diagnostic X-ray indicates all except d. and e.

Treatment: if causing symptoms need removal surgically.

OSGOOD-SCHLATTER'S DISEASE is common in 12-15 year-olds, due to traction on the tibial tubercle by the insertion of the patellar tendon. May be bilateral. Adolescents complaining of a dull ache in this region with a tender-lump should be X-rayed.

Treatment: usually resolves with several weeks rest, but may need P.O.P. for up to 8 weeks.

RUPTURE OF THE QUADRICEPS TENDON, PATELLAR LIGAMENT, OR RECTUS FEMORIS needs operative repair. Extension at the knee is painful and poor (see lig. injury).

BURSAE are common around the knee, PREPATELLAR bursitis (housemaid's knee) is a swelling on the anterior aspect of the patella, is rounded and fluctuant. INFRAPATELLAR bursitis (clergyman's knee) is a swelling over the insertion of the patella tendon. Tenderness of the patella tendon (PATELLAR TENDINITIS) may be seen in footballers after repeatedly kicking a ball (shooting practice).

SEMIMEMBRANOSUS bursa occurs between this muscle and the medial head of gastrocnemius. It presents as a painless lump behind the knee, more obvious when extended, and there is NO expression of fluid into the knee joint. BAKER'S CYST

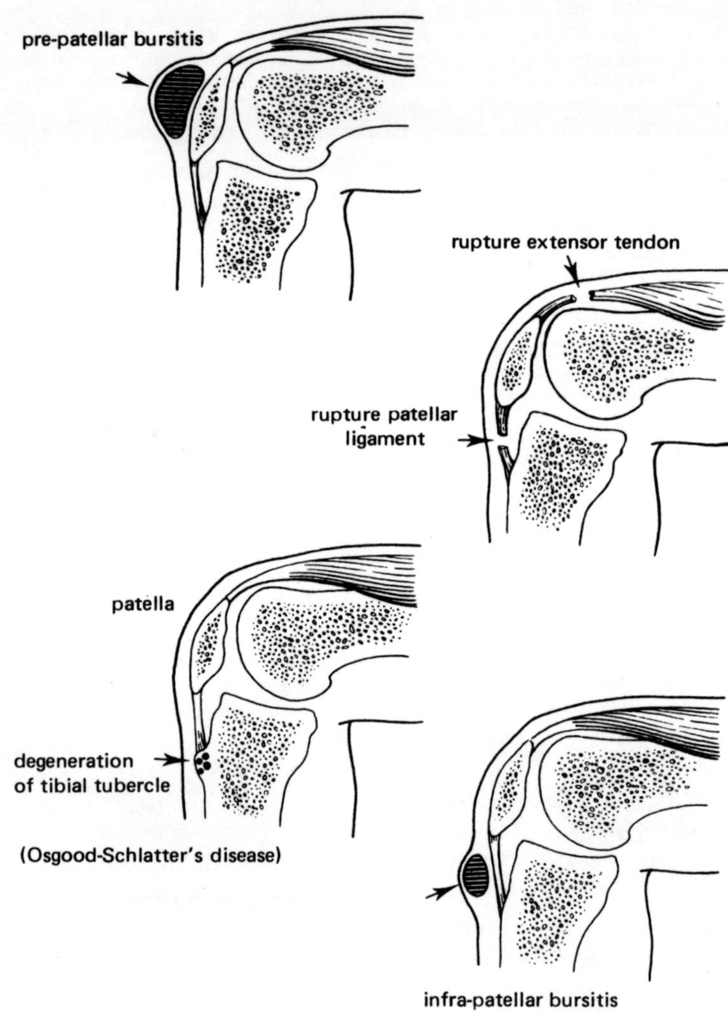

Illustration showing injury points around knee

presents as a fluctuant lump in the midline posteriorly at joint level: since it communicates with the joint it can be expressed. The underlying cause is mild osteoarthritis and accompanying effusion that herniates through the posterior capsule of the joint. All except Baker's cyst can be aspirated and a pressure dressing applied. Baker's cysts are treated by a reduction in activity or rest so that the osteoarthritic process subsides and the effusion becomes reduced.

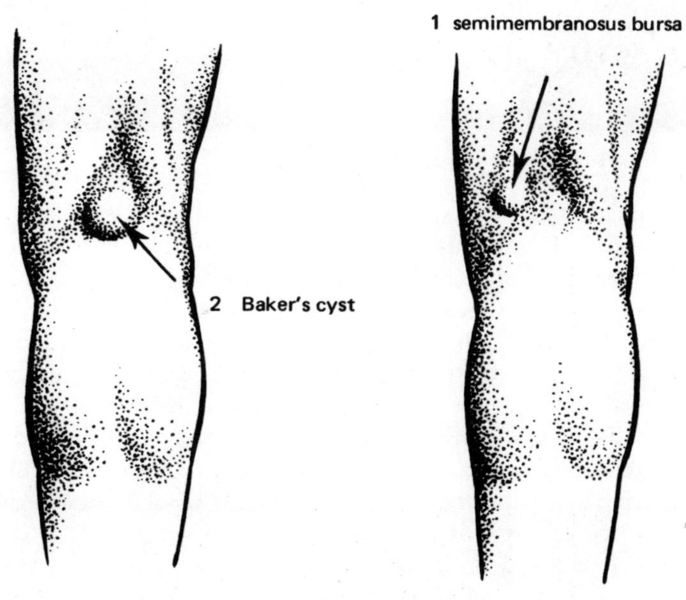

Illustration showing swellings behind knee

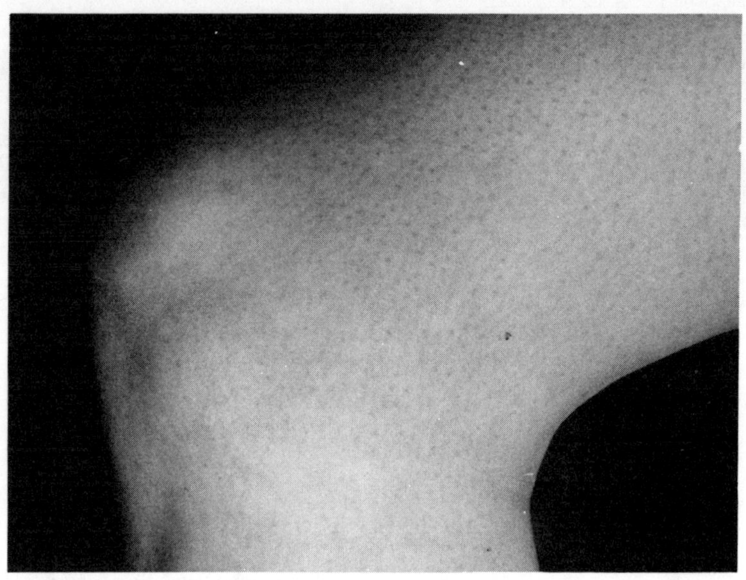

Photograph showing cyst of lateral cartilage at knee

Cysts of the EXTERNAL CARTILAGE (see later) have to be differentiated from bursae. Calcification in the medial ligament (called malady of Pellegrini-Stieda) may be occasionally seen on X-ray, due to repeated minor tears. Usually settles with rest. In SKI-ING the knee and ankle are regularly sprained. The medial ligament of the knee is commonly damaged, especially a partial tear of the deep fibres. Ankle injuries are almost always rotational, any of the ligaments can be damaged, and fractures of either internal or external malleoli are common. In novice skiers the commonest mechanism of injury is due to divergence of the skis or crossing the skis on a tow. With the more experienced skier catching an outside edge when turning or an inside edge when traversing causes the damage. The ski becomes fixed but the body continues at speed, then the Achilles' tendon might be torn.

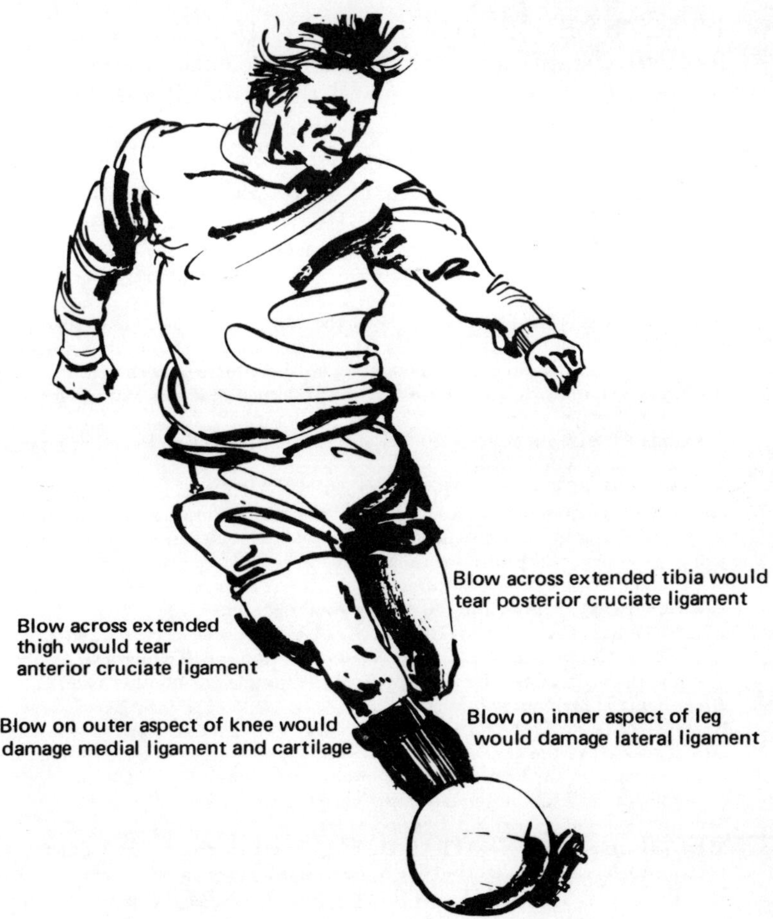
Blow across extended tibia would tear posterior cruciate ligament
Blow across extended thigh would tear anterior cruciate ligament
Blow on outer aspect of knee would damage medial ligament and cartilage
Blow on inner aspect of leg would damage lateral ligament

Injuries to the Leg

The leg consists of two bones, the tibia and fibula, of which the former is much the larger and more important, since it is the main weight-bearing bone of the leg. Fractures may occur independently or together.

FRACTURE OF THE TIBIA AND FIBULA. A twisting force to a stationary foot or direct violence causes a fracture of both. Great pain ensues and the deformity and tenderness is easily felt, since both are subcutaneous.

Treatment: reduction under general anaesthetic and P.O.P. for 6–12 weeks. Unstable fractures may need plating and screwing.

FRACTURES OF THE TIBIA are treated as above.

FRACTURES OF THE FIBULA cause tenderness over the bone but if they do not involve the stability of the ankle joint they can be treated by a crepe bandage or strapping for 3 weeks.

STRESS FRACTURES occur in both the tibia (one type of shin soreness) and fibula due to prolonged road work and repeated minor trauma to the shaft of the bone. A dull aching pain is complained of by the athlete over the bone concerned. An X-ray will indicate the fracture by the periosteal reaction, but not for 4 weeks. A localised tender area may be found in the bone.

Treatment: rest from activity for 3–4 weeks. Then reduction in activity, protective footwear (thick soled shoes).

ANTERIOR TIBIAL COMPARTMENT SYNDROME is due to overuse of the anterior tibial muscles in running (shin soreness of long distance runners) and soccer, resulting in muscle swelling within the fascia. Occasionally pain is referred along the course of the anterior tibial nerve, which is compressed, onto the dorsum of the foot. With extreme swelling patchy areas of muscle necrosis are found.

Treatment: rest and elevation to relieve swelling.

PULLED GASTROCNEMIUS (or SOLEUS) occurs after sudden propulsion forwards, accompanied by pain and weakness in the calf. Tenderness, swelling and a lump appear in either the main belly of the muscle or on either head.

Treatment: as for muscle injury.

RUPTURED PLANTARIS. This is a very small muscle which arises from the lateral condyle of the knee and runs down the medial aspect of the Achilles tendon to its insertion in the heel. It is occasionally torn (tennis leg). Mild pain or aching of sudden onset is felt on the outer aspect of the leg.

Treatment: none needed but a period of rest.

MULTIPLE SUBPERIOSTEAL HAEMATOMAS give an irregular feel to the anterior surface of the tibia but are of no importance (footballer's shin).

RUPTURE OF THE ACHILLES TENDON may be partial or complete, leading to loss of propulsion. This injury occurs suddenly and pulls the athlete up in his tracks, causing him/her to limp to the touch line. If complete, a palpable gap above the

FRACTURES OF TIBIA AND FIBULA

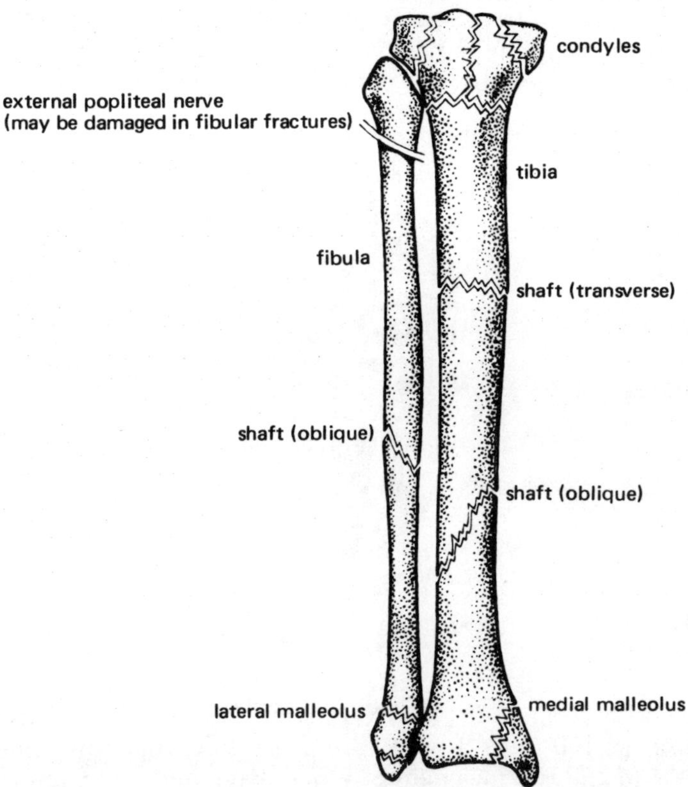

heel is detected. This complete tear requires suture and P.O.P. for 6 or more weeks. Partial ruptures are treated with rest, but may need suture or P.O.P. if large. PERITENDINITIS, common in middle distance runners, responds to heat and physiotherapy (see injuries of tendons).
N.B. Even in complete rupture of the Achilles tendon there is some movement (plantar flexion) of the foot due to the action of accessory muscles (tibialis post. and peroneus longus).

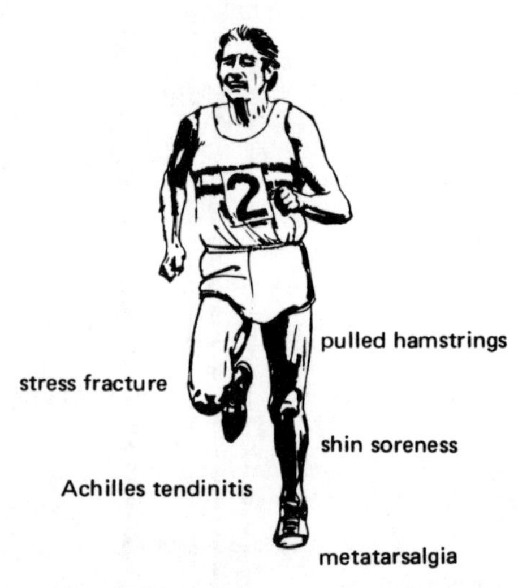

ATHLETES, especially LONG DISTANCE RUNNERS who do over 100 miles a week, are prone to chronic muscular disorders in the the lower limb. Once diagnosed, then immediate reduction in activity, to rest, support and elevation is mandatory with a gradual build-up to full activity. Muscle injuries CANNOT be run off, prevention is by warming up the body with track suit and gentle jogging and exercises before an event, and thick rubber soled shoes for prolonged road work.

Injuries to the Ankle

SPRAINS are common in athletes. The ankle joint has many tough, but short, ligaments associated with it, thickened on the inner and outer side to form the medial and lateral ligaments; the former being attached to the tibia, the latter to the fibula. Movements of the TALUS within the ankle joint are found in conjunction with mobility in the joint between the talus and calcaneus (the SUBTALAR JOINT). Movements at the subtalar joint are called inversion (adduction) and eversion (abduction) of the foot. Thus SPRAINS of the 'ankle' may be due to stretching of soft tissues in either the ankle joint proper or the subtalar joints. Both joints can be stabilised with strapping, permitting activity with MINOR sprains.

With partial or complete tears in the medial, lateral, deltoid, and interosseus ligaments prolonged strapping or P.O.P. may be used for 2–4 weeks.

FRACTURES . . . occur in the ankle in a bewildering variety, depending on the direction of deforming force, and whether both bones are damaged, and whether the talus is dislocated.

FRACTURE OF THE LATERAL MALLEOLUS. If minor or above the joint line these can be strapped for 3 weeks. If joint stability is threatened, however, P.O.P. 3–5 weeks.

FRACTURES OF THE MEDIAL MALLEOLUS usually lead to joint instability due to involvement of the medial and deltoid ligaments.

Treatment: P.O.P. 4–6 weeks. May need screw fixation.

POTT'S FRACTURE is a FRACTURE/DISLOCATION of the ankle which needs accurate reduction and fixation. The true Pott's fracture is due to a force directed laterally that first of all fractures the lateral malleolus (from the inside out), then tears the ligaments on the medial side of the ankle often tearing a chip off the medial malleolus, and finally pushing the talus backwards to fracture the posterior surface of the tibia and tear the joint capsule. Gross pain and swelling accompany such an injury and the deformity is obvious. (Common in ski-ing).

Treatment: reduction under general anaesthetic. P.O.P. for 8–12 weeks. May need screws and pins.

TENDINITIS OR TENOSYNOVITIS AROUND THE ANKLE. The tendons around the ankle become puffy and

INJURIES AT ANKLE
(varieties of Pott's fracture)

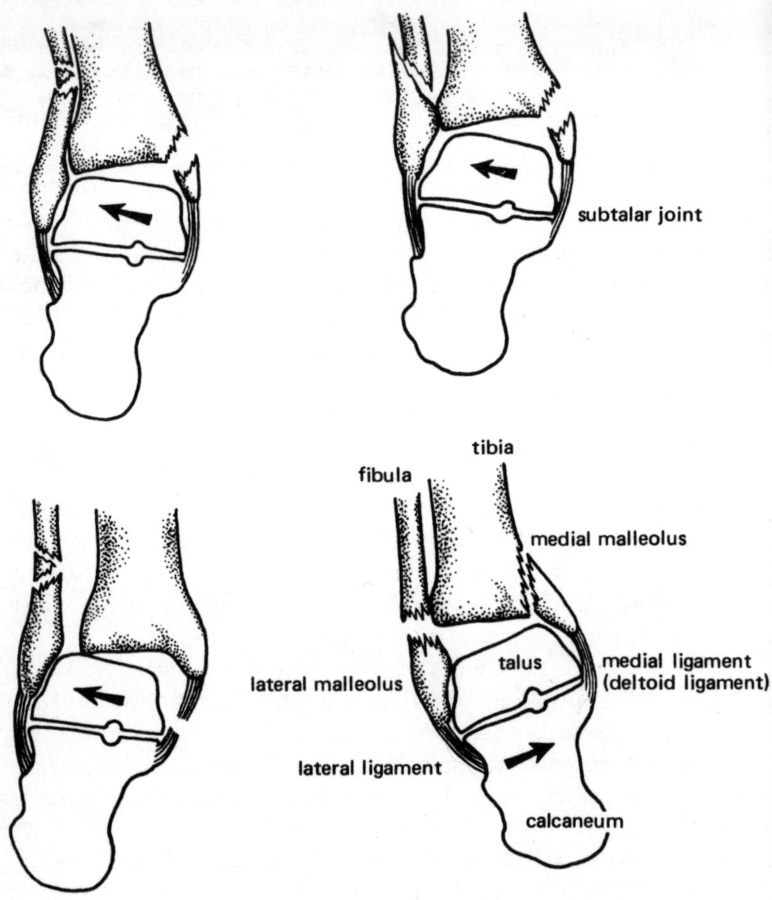

arrow shows direction of force

Injuries at ankle
classical Pott's fracture
Foot dislocated backwards

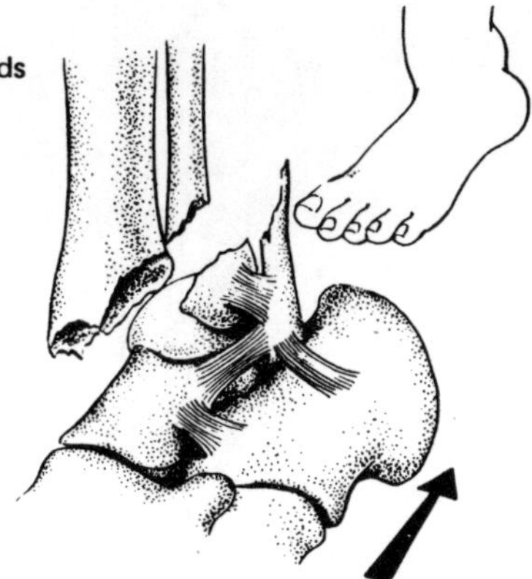

swollen due to swelling in their sheaths, especially after overuse. Occasionally the retaining ligaments (retinaculum) become torn or stretched.

Treatment: rest, heat, physiotherapy, and sometimes steroids and ultrasound.

FOOTBALLER'S ANKLE is due to repeated small tears in the anterior aspect of the ankle joint from dead-ball kicking and shooting. The many capsular scars produced become calcified and small spicules of bone are found at the insertion of the joint capsule into the bone. The player usually complains of a dull aching pain around the ankle, worse after the above activities.

Treatment: rest, heat, physiotherapy, manipulation, and occasionally operative removal of bony spicules.

An EFFUSION within the ankle joint cannot be recognised from the anterior aspect because of the many structures passing over it, but when viewed from behind a fullness is seen in the retromalleolar fossae.

In FOOTBALL the ankle is particularly vulnerable from sliding tackles or 'clash of feet', sprains are especially common, and often the anterior fibres of the lateral ligament are torn, with tenderness and swelling over the anterior aspect of the lateral malleolus. The posterior and middle fibres of the same ligament may be torn when the opposing player's boot comes through in a tackle from behind.

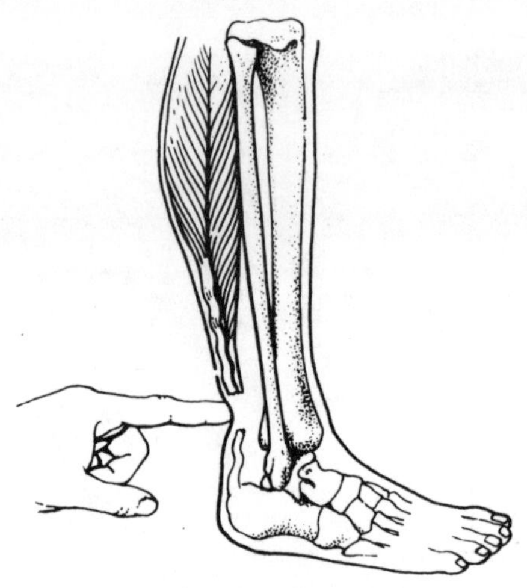

Ruptured Achilles tendon

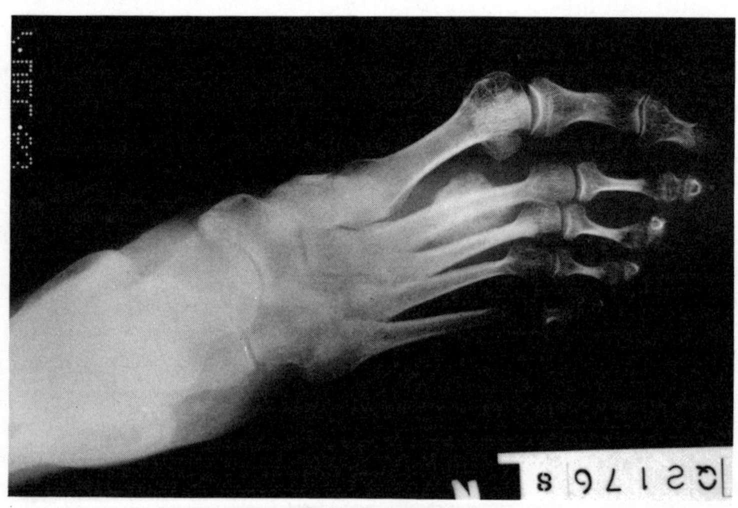

Xray showing March fracture (2nd metatarsal)

Injuries to the Foot

The many small bones of the foot, tarsal, metatarsal and phalanges, are connected by a maze of ligaments and tendon-insertions which can be damaged or torn.
FRACTURES of the larger bones require rest and P.O.P. for several weeks, but fractures of the metatarsals and phalanges may only need strapping, usually take 3–4 weeks for union.
FRACTURES OF THE CALCANEUM are the most important, commonly due to a fall from a height on to the heel. The are serious when they involve the subtalar joint, when operative fixation and reduction may be necessary with P.O.P. 6–12 weeks. Otherwise treated by padding, crepe and elevation, to unite within 12 weeks.
STRESS FRACTURES are found after overactivity, e.g. road walking and running and usually involve the 2nd metatarsal head. Pain is found on the sole of the foot over the affected bone.
Treatment: rest, occasionally P.O.P.
METATARSALGIA is pain over the metatarsal heads, may be due to stress fracture, ligamentous strain (flat foot), or a bulbous swelling of the nerves (MORTON'S NEUROMA).
FLAT FOOT may be congenital, due to previous multiple fractures, chronic foot strain, or spasm of the peroneal muscles.
Treatment: physiotherapy and foot strengthening exercises.
PLANTAR FASCIITIS causes a dull aching pain in the region of the heel on the sole of the foot, and is due to chronic irritation from repeated trauma, e.g. fast bowlers, hurdlers, long jumpers etc., in the plantar fascia that ensheaths and protects the sole. Often a small spicule of bone develops at the insertion of fascia in the calcaneum (spur).
Treatment: rest, padding, physiotherapy, steroid injections and occasionally operation.
GANGLION is a small tense swelling over the dorsum of the foot (may be found at the wrist). It feels like an extra bone, and is caused by small ligament degeneration.
Treatment: excision.
HALLUX VALGUS, HALLUX RIGIDUS, HAMMER TOE . . . Hallux valgus is due to the great toe being forced outwards by an ill fitting boot or shoe: ultimately a bursa (bunion) forms from friction. Hallux rigidus is due to arthritic changes in the first metatarso-phalangeal joint, the main complaint being pain and stiffness. Hammer toe is an easily recognisable deformity of the toes due to ligamentous or tendon contracture.
Treatment: all need surgical correction.
SUBUNGUAL HAEMATOMA causes great pain and can be relieved quite simply by boring a hole in the nail over the blood clot with a sterile needle.
INGROWING TOE NAIL is caused by the great toe nail being pressed by ill-fitting shoes into the skin of the toe causing infection and granulation tissue. Padding may relieve this condition in its early stages but removal of the nail may be required.
BLISTERS are the curse of the pre-season training. Small blisters can be covered

with an adhesive dressing. Larger ones are burst with a sterile needle and dressed. Boots and shoes should be checked for friction points, new stiff leather needs running in gradually.
Treatment: as above. Surgical spirit or mercurochrome can be used to dry up weeping surfaces and harden skin.

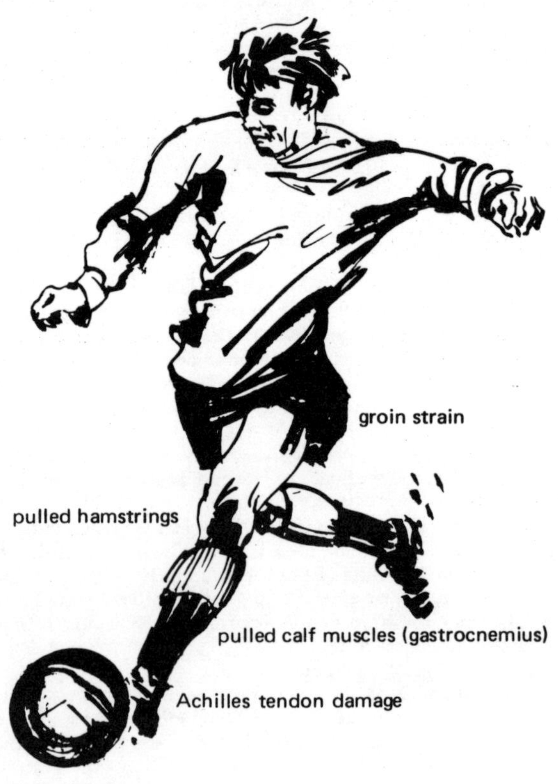

Perfect balance and muscle tone prevents injuries and improves mobility and performance

3. THE STRUCTURE OF THE BODY
(Anatomy and Histology)

THE SKIN is the sensitive covering of the body that conserves the moisture of the underlying tissues, regulates temperature by radiation and evaporation (sweating), and protects us against the external environment, notably invading germs.

It consists of two parts . . . the EPIDERMIS, made up of five horizontal layers of cells.
. . . the DERMIS, a connective tissue layer with vessels and nerves.

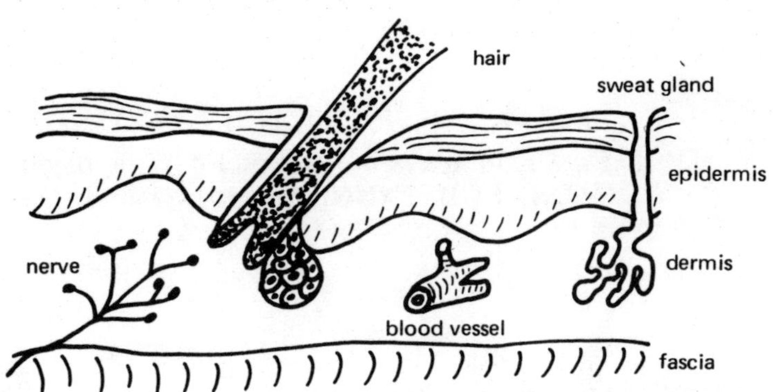

Section through upper layers of skin

The EPIDERMIS is rapidly repaired from the basal layer of cells, partial damage of this nature constitutes an abrasion.

With damage to the DERMIS the small vessels bleed and the elastic fibres produce gaping of the skin edges. Thus sutures are necessary.

The skin has natural creases and whorls due to the arrangement of the connective tissue of the dermis, called Lange's lines. These must be approximated to minimise scar tissue formation.

The boundary between epidermis and dermis is not evenly horizontal, but thrown into ridges called dermal papillae. Special nerve endings, found in the folds, are distorted by pressure, enhancing tactile sensitivity. There are 312 hairs per square centimetre, with their accompanying sebaceous glands that oil the skin and protects it from drying and germs. Removal of sebaceous fluid by repeated washing, prolonged bandaging or plaster of paris leads to excessive flaking and infection. There are 120 sweat glands per sq. cm. that produce a dilute salty secretion. With prolonged sweating the body becomes depleted in salt and water and cramps and giddiness ensue. The nails are a modification of the clear layer, and grow at the rate of $1\frac{1}{2}''$ per year. Damage to a wide area of skin, if not sutured, heals by granulation tissue (proud flesh) leading to a long period of incapacity and an ugly scar.

CONNECTIVE TISSUE is the packing tissue in the body and serves a multiplicity of functions. A thorough understanding of this substance is essential for all concerned with sports injuries, for it is the basic component of the locomotor system.

CONNECTIVE TISSUE consists of

FIBRES, collagen, elastic, and reticular (immature collagen).

..CELLS, fibroblasts that produce the fibres, and other cells that are modified white corpuscles of the blood.

..the GROUND SUBSTANCE which surrounds the cells and fibres.

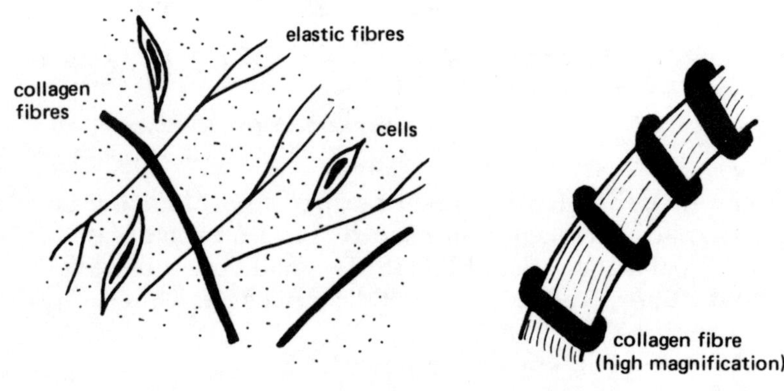

Connective tissue (high magnification)

COLLAGEN FIBRES are exceedingly strong but inelastic. Arranged in sheets or bundles they form TENDONS, LIGAMENTS, the CAPSULE of JOINTS, APONEUROSIS, and INTERMUSCULAR FASCIA. Thus these structures all have the same response to injury, and when torn heal by SCAR TISSUE, which is an irregularly arranged collagen formation. Usually scars regain only 70% of the normal strength of the regularly arranged collagen, and are a potential weak point in the tendon or ligament etc. concerned. Blood clots (haematoma) in the tissues of the body are converted into scar tissues and form adhesions that stick muscle groups together and bind down ligaments and tendons. Massage and hydrocortisone breaks down these adhesions, heat aids their reabsorption, and evacuation of clots limits their formation.

Alteration in the consistency of the ground substance produces CARTILAGE, known as fibrocartilage when fibres are present. The hyaline cartilage of joints is devoid of fibres. Damage to cartilage from trauma leads to cracking, fibrillation, and detachment of small pieces that can cause locking in a joint. Cartilage heals badly for it is devoid of blood vessels. Excessive cartilaginous damage is the precursor to osteoarthritis in a joint. The deposition of calcium, phosphate and other substances in cartilage forms BONE.

The 'cartilages' of the knee are special moon-shaped structures that allow increased mobility. They are made up of fibrocartilage and being avascular do not heal after tearing, unless the tear is at the periphery close to the capsule of the joint. They occasionally regrow after surgical removal. Torn menisci ('cartilages' in the knee) need removing for they promote ligamentous stretching and later osteoarthritis. Articular discs ('cartilages') are found in the joints of the jaw, sternoclavicular, acromioclavicular and inferior radio-ulnar as well as the knee-joints.

JOINTS. A joint or articulation is formed when two bones meet one another. They are divided into FIBROUS, CARTILAGINOUS and SYNOVIAL.

FIBROUS joints occur when bones are fastened together with fibrous tissue, as in the skull suture lines. No movement is possible.

CARTILAGINOUS joints have the opposed bony surfaces connected to each other by cartilage and a limited amount of movement is permitted. Such articulations are found between the vertebral bodies in the spine and in the pelvis at the symphysis.

SYNOVIAL JOINTS. These are the moving joints of the body, including all articulations in the limbs. They contain SYNOVIAL FLUID, secreted by a SYNOVIAL MEMBRANE, hence their name. This fluid is contained in the joint cavity and surrounded by the joint capsule. It also bathes the hyaline cartilage at the ends of the long bone, producing a system five times as slippery as ice on ice. Thus in order to maintain an upright balance the capsule is thickened into ligaments that prevent excessive movement.

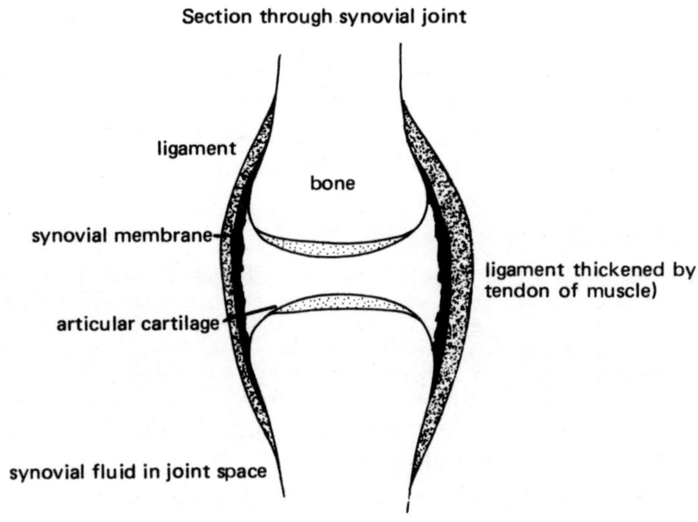

The tendons of muscles that cross the external surface of a joint also limit mobility. When damaged the synovial membrane pours out fluid or blood, depending on the severity of the injury. With rest this effusion will be absorbed. Excessive blood in a joint (haemarthrosis) forms adhesions and needs aspiration in a hospital. Infections within a joint cause gross damage to the structures, especially the cartilage, and need prompt treatment in bed with antibiotics.

The following movements are found in a synoval joint. Flexion or bending, extension or straightening, adduction—a movement towards the midline, abduction —away from body, internal rotation and external rotation (see diagram).
Joints are sometimes classified into hinge joints (elbow e.g.), plane or flat joints (e.g. wrist), ball- and -socket (hip, shoulder), condyloid (base of finger), saddle (base of thumb at wrist) and pivot (head of the radius at the elbow).

MEASURING AND RECORDING JOINT FUNCTION

General Principles

1. All movement should be measured by degrees from a neutral point of zero.
2. The neutral point from which the movement is measured must be defined, if possible.
3. It is always worth while to observe the comparative movement in the joint of the opposite limb.
4. Angles should be measured with a goniometer and protractor.
5. The range of movement in the joints above and below the affected part should be measured.
6. Never force a joint into an abnormal position.
7. The production of pain indicates damage is being done—stop immediately.

MOVEMENTS AT SHOULDER

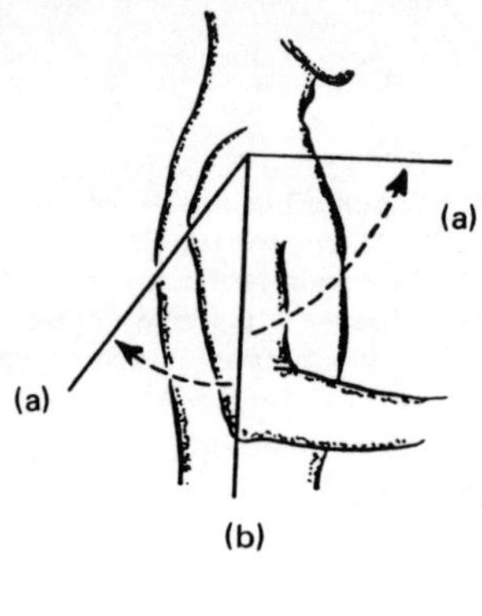

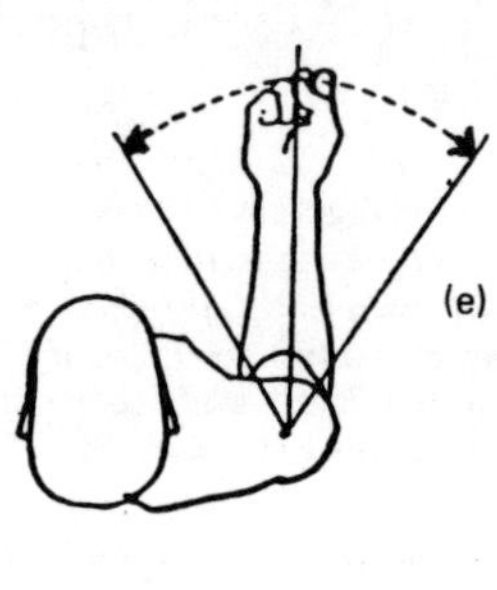

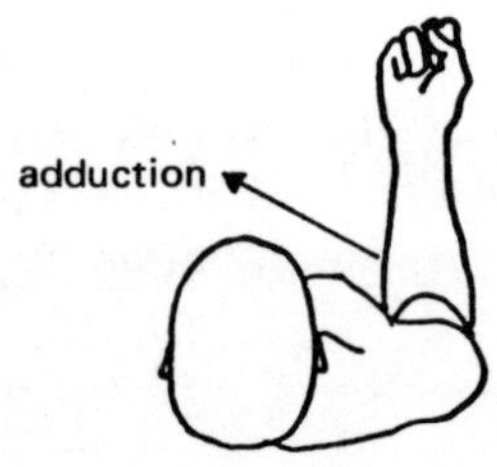

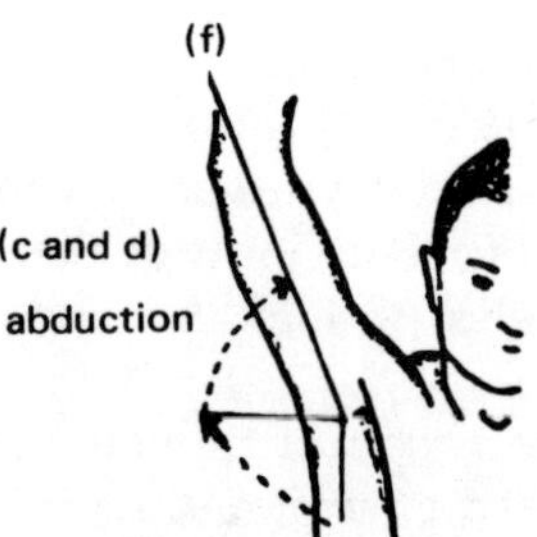

Shoulder movements. *Neutral position* is arm to side, elbow flexed to 90°, forearm pointing forward. a, *Flexion* and *extension.* b, *Neutral.* c, *Abduction*—maximum 90°. d, *Rotation in abduction.* e, *Rotation in neutral* (arm behind back to test extreme internal rotation—compared with opposite side). f, *Elevation*—compared with opposite side and measured in number of degrees. (This is shoulder-girdle motion as compared with items a to e, which are true humeroscapular motions.)

MOVEMENTS OF SPINE

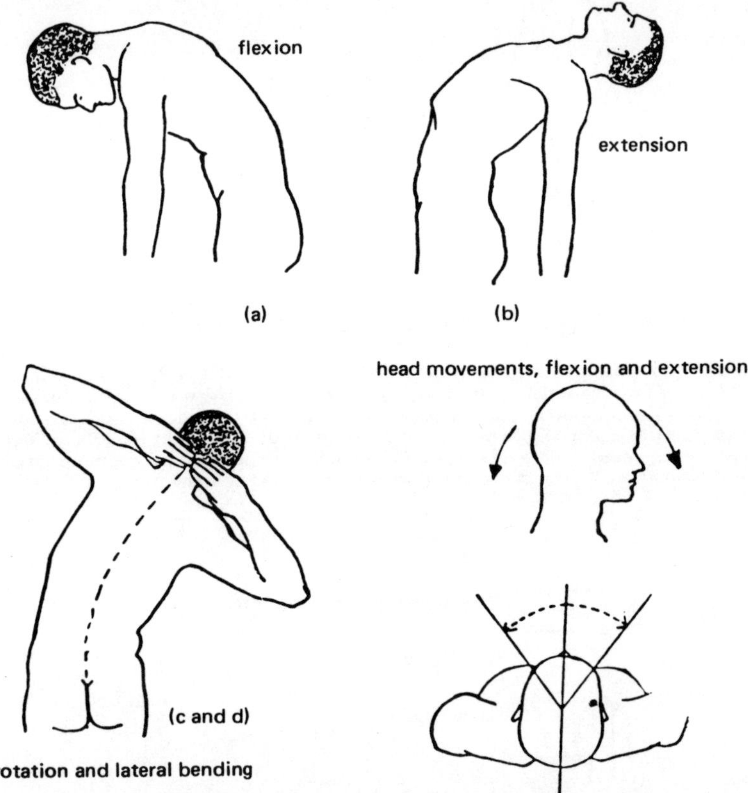

Spinal movements. *Neutral position* cannot be defined. a, *Forward bending*—this motion cannot be measured accurately in degrees, but should be compared with the probable normal for the age of the patient. It should be noted whether the lumbar spine flattens itself or reverses itself. Motions should be carried out in both sitting and standing positions. b, *Extension*—it should be noted to what degree the dorsal and lumbar curves change. c, *Lateral bending*—right and left. d, *Rotation* with pelvis fixed—right and left, comparing angle the shoulders make with pelvis.

Neck movements. *Neutral position* is with head up and chin in. *Rotation*—right and left. *Flexion and extension. Lateral bending*—right and left.

ELBOW AND FINGER MOVEMENTS

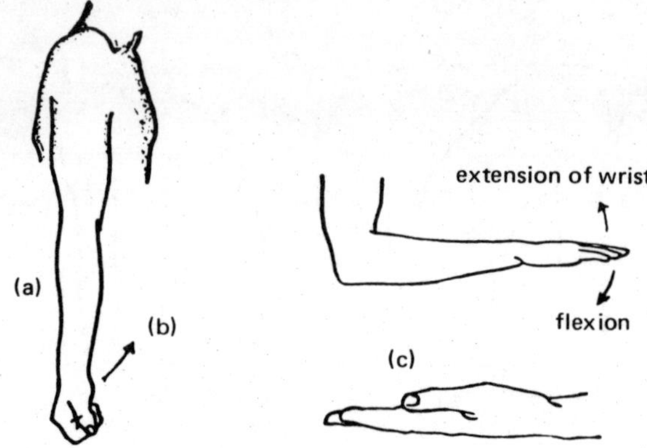

Elbow movements. a, *Neutral position* is with forearm in extension. b, *Flexion*—measured from complete extension, the neutral point. *Hyperextension* measured in degrees as compared with the opposite elbow. When there is loss of complete extension, this loss should be recorded in degrees of permanent flexion. c, *Supination* (palm up) from a neutral point—which is midposition between pronation and supination. *Pronation* (palm down)—elbow must be fixed at side in 90° of flexion.

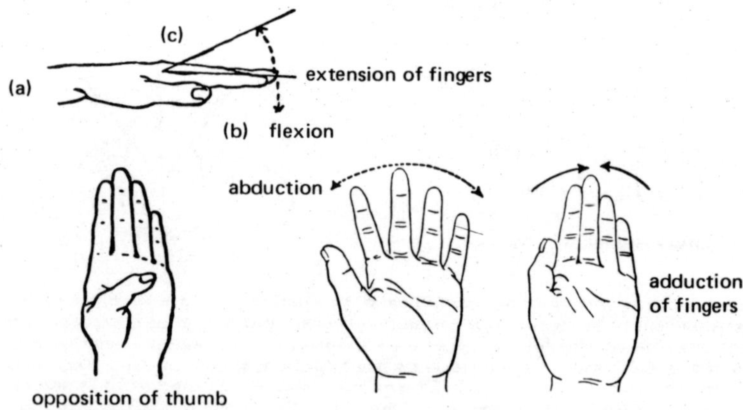

Finger movements. a, *Neutral position* is with fingers in extension. b, All motions are in *flexion* either in the metacarpophalangeal or interphalangeal joints. c, *Hyperextension* should be noted if present. d, *Abduction* and *adduction.* Test should be made for increased lateral mobility.

HIP MOVEMENTS

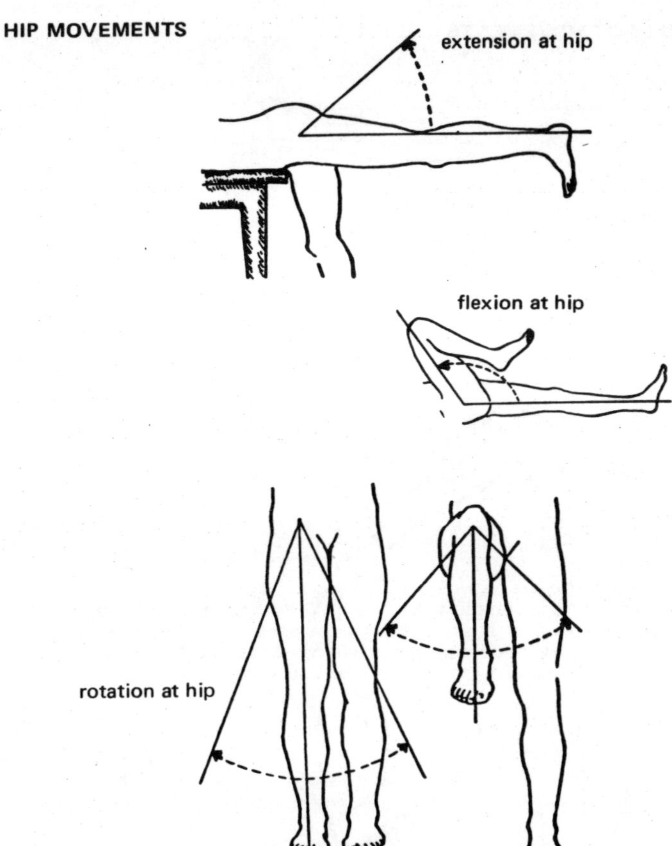

Hip movements. a, *Neutral position* is with hip in extension, patella pointing upward. b, *Flexion* is measured with the knee bent, and the opposite thigh must remain in neutral. c, To test *permanent flexion,* the opposite thigh must be flexed, so as to flatten the lumbar spine and to fix the pelvis. d, *Hyperextension*—neutral, the same as for flexion, but with the patient lying prone with opposite thigh over the end of table at an angle of 90°. e, *Rotation* (external and internal) *in extension.* Measurement should be made with patient prone and knee flexed to 90°. f, *Abduction*—measured from a line which forms an angle of 90° with a line joining the anterosuperior spines. *Adduction*—the same. g, *Rotation* (external and internal) *in flexion.* Measurement should be made with patient on back with knee and thigh flexed to 90° angles.

KNEE AND FOOT MOVEMENTS

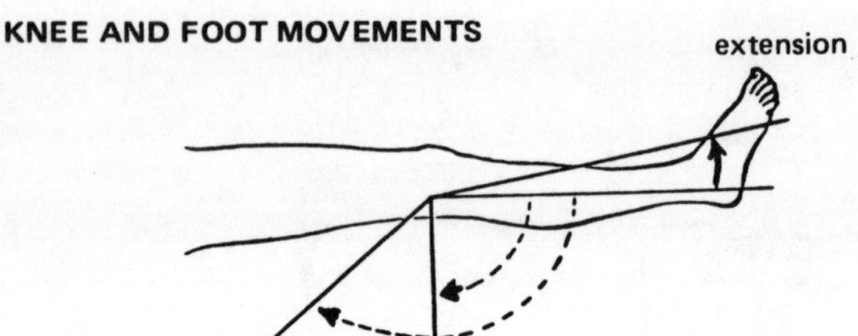

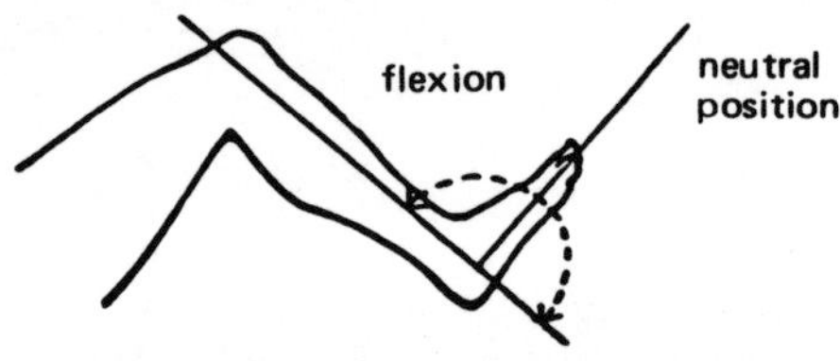

Knee movements. a, *Neutral position* is with complete extension. b, *Flexion*—measured in degrees from complete extension. When there is loss of complete extension, it should be recorded in degrees of permanent flexion. *Hyperextension. Anteroposterior* stablility should be tested with the knee at 90° flexion. *Lateral stability* should be tested with the knee in complete extension.

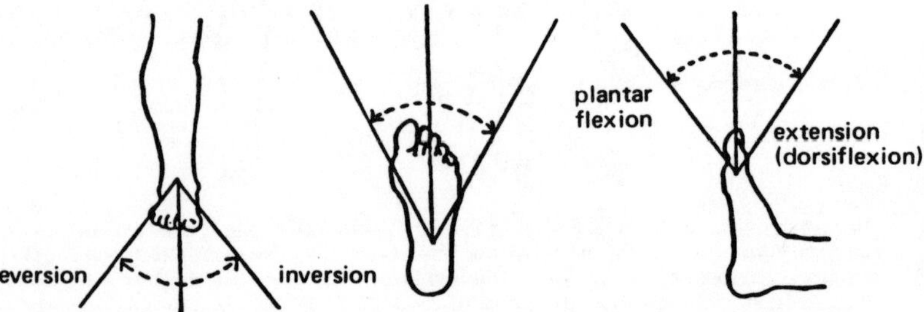

Ankle movements. a, *Neutral position* is with the angle made by the outer border of the foot and the leg at 90° and in neutral with regard to inversion and eversion. b, *Dorsiflexion* should be tested with the foot in inversion. Measurements should be compared with knee flexed and with knee in extension to rule out tight calf muscles. *Plantar flexion* should be measured in degrees from neutral position.

MUSCLE. The property of contractility is highly developed in muscle, and once the delicate fibres are destroyed they *cannot* be replaced.

Muscles are of three types:

SMOOTH or INvoluntary, a primitive form found in the bowel, lungs and all other organs, contracts automatically.

..CARDIAC, only found in the heart, contracts rhythmically, has striped fibres.

..VOLUNTARY or STRIPED MUSCLE, the muscle of locomotion.

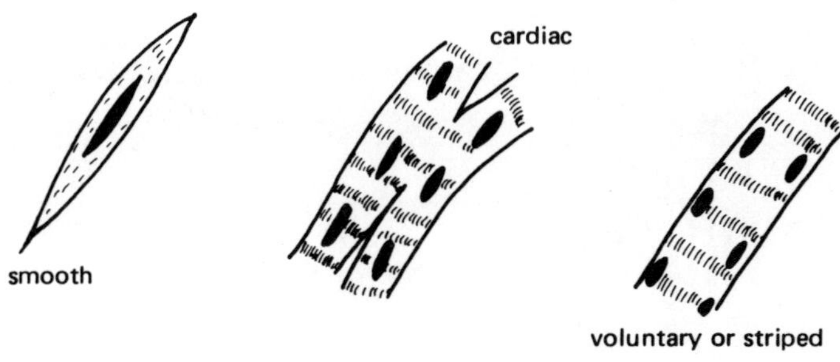

Types of muscle fibre

Voluntary muscle consists of fibres (10μ–100μ) bound together in a matrix of connective tissue. Unlike cardiac muscle, these fibres do not branch. The surface of each fibre is covered by a thin membrane, the sarcolemma, within each fibre are many nuclei (unlike other tissue-cells). Fibres have a striped appearance, these bands are the A (dark) and I (light) bands, and are produced by the arrangement of proteins (actin and mysoin) within the fibre. During a contraction strands of these proteins interdigitate and the muscle length is shortened but the volume remains almost unchanged (slightly less).

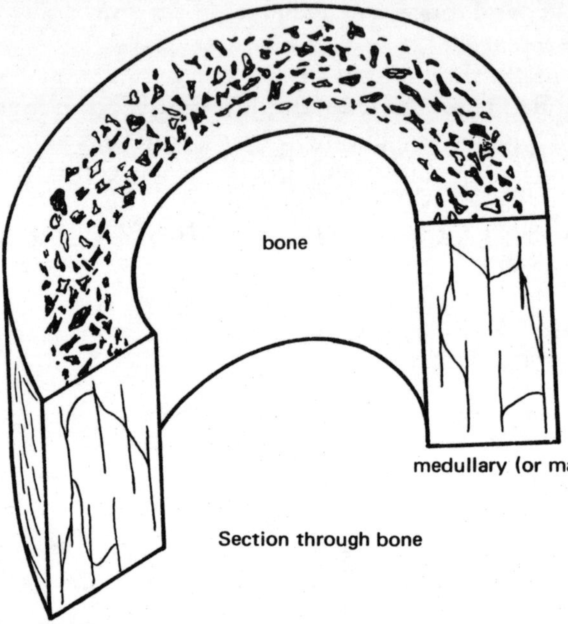

bone
medullary (or marrow) cavity
cortex (with Haversian canals)

Section through bone

tendon
periosteum

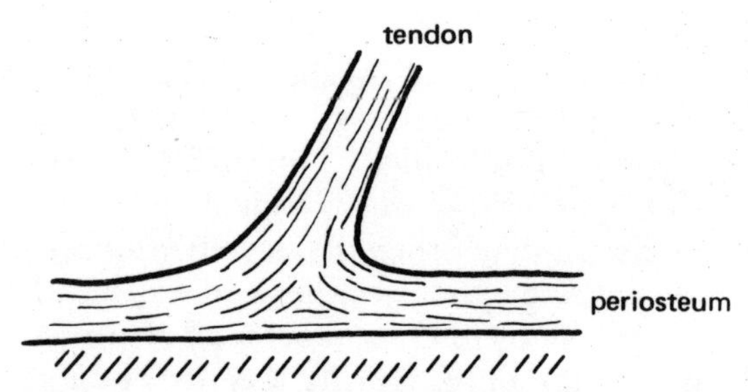

insertion of tendon or ligament into periosteum

Each fibre has a delicate covering outside the sarcolemma called an endomysium and is bound into bundles by the perimysium. Finally all the bundles are covered by the epimysium which coats the muscle and becomes thickened to form intra-muscular septa. After injury blood tracks along these septa. under the influencc of gravity and contraction and thus appears at sites distant to the point of original injury.

The muscle fibres end bluntly in a tendon, the direct continuation of the connective tissues (endo- and perimysium) into the fibres of the tendon constitutes the connection. Tears occur at this junction, which is a relative weak point. Muscles shorten to about 65% of their length (isotonic, for the tone remains unchanged). When the muscle contracts but does not shorten, e.g. when pressing against a wall, the contraction is isometric.

NO MUSCLE EVER ACTS ALONE. The prime mover initiates the action aided by the synergists (the helpers), and movement can only occur if the antagonistic muscles relax. Complex nervous reflexes co-ordinate such contractions, these are heightened by practice and constitute skills of the sport concerned. Nerves produce contraction by passing a minute electrical current into the muscle (40 mV) and activating the proteins mentioned above.

BONES. The general framework of the body is built up mainly of a series of bones, supplemented in certain regions by cartilage. Bones provide the central axis and give form to the tissues, protect the brain and chest, provide a system of levers for locomotion and afford areas for the attachment of muscles. Bones are of four types, Long, Short, Flat and Pneumatic (as the bones of the face with sinuses). Each bone has a shaft or body surrounding a marrow cavity, in which the blood elements are formed. During the growing period (up to 20 years) there are one or more cartilagenous discs in each bone—the EPIPHYSEAL CARTILAGE, from which the bone grows, and through which fractures occur (called displaced epiphysis). Damage to these special areas may result in a complete cessation of growth, and ultimate limb shortening. The bones are surrounded by PERIOSTEUM, a fine connective tissue skin, which contains most of the vessels and nerves, and also the small cells (osteoblasts) that remodel the osseous tissue after a fracture. Blood clots under the periosteum are known as subperiosteal haematomas. They may be converted into bony lumps or nodules that characterise a footballer's shin.

Periosteum covers the bone up to the articular cartilage. It gives attachment to the ligaments, tendons, muscles etc.

The surface of a bone has many variable features, which are given special descriptive terms. A condyle is a smooth round elevation, an epicondyle is an elevation above the condyle, smooth or rough projections on the shaft are called a tubercle or tuberosity, a trochlea is a pulley-shaped surface, a hamulus a hook, a cornu a horn-like process, a distinct ridge is a crest, a very narrow one becomes a line (linea). A hole in a bone is known as a foramen, a bony tunnel a canal, a groove is called a sulcus, a notch an incisure, a gap a hiatus, a thin plate a lamina. Depressions are described as fossae.

The insertion of a tendon, ligament or muscle into a bone usually results in a surface elevation or depression.

Bones show clearly on X-ray, but small fractures, especially of long standing, are only indicated by a reaction in the periosteum which becomes thickened over the fracture line (the periosteal or cortical reaction).

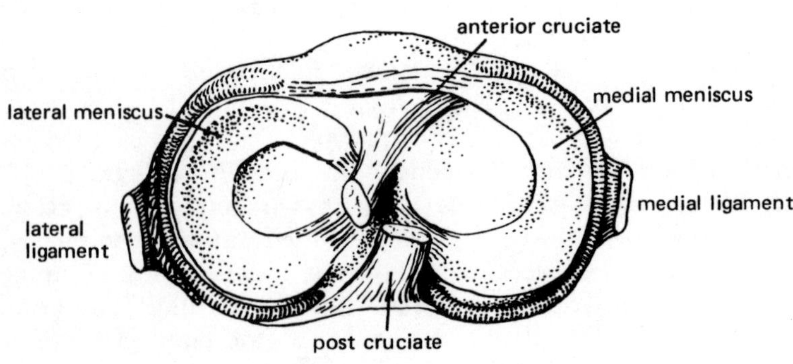

Knee joint from above (femur removed)

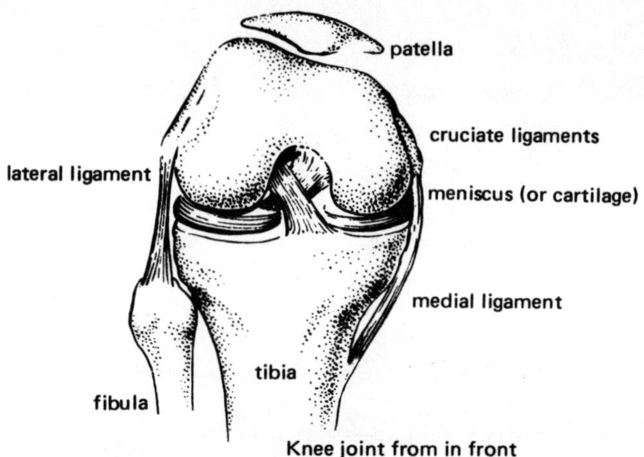

Knee joint from in front

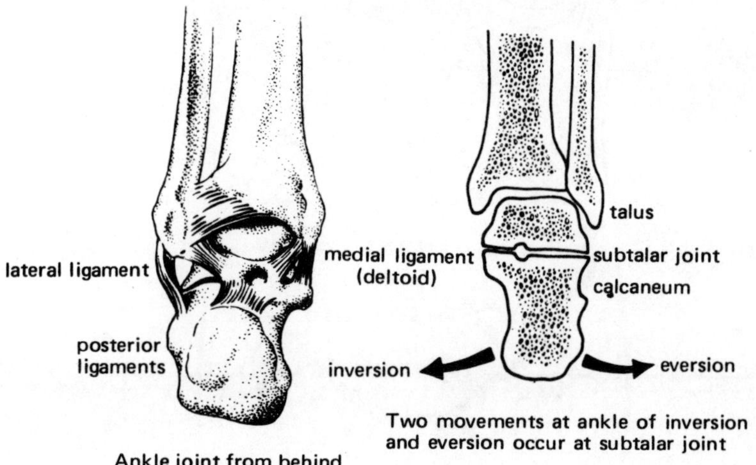

Two movements at ankle of inversion and eversion occur at subtalar joint

Ankle joint from behind

CHEST AND ABDOMEN (anterior)

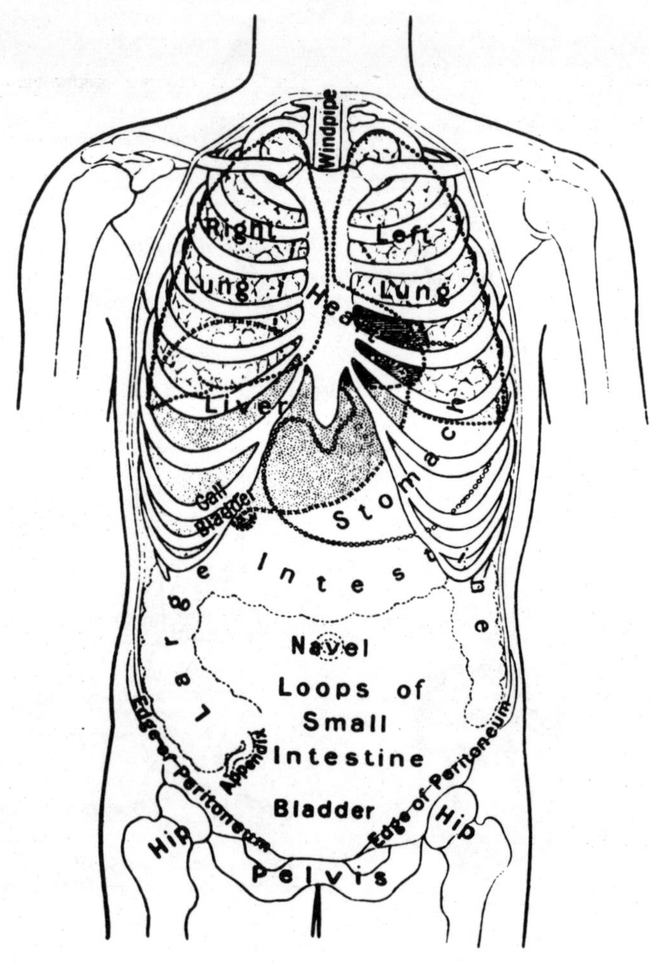

CHEST AND ABDOMEN (posterior)

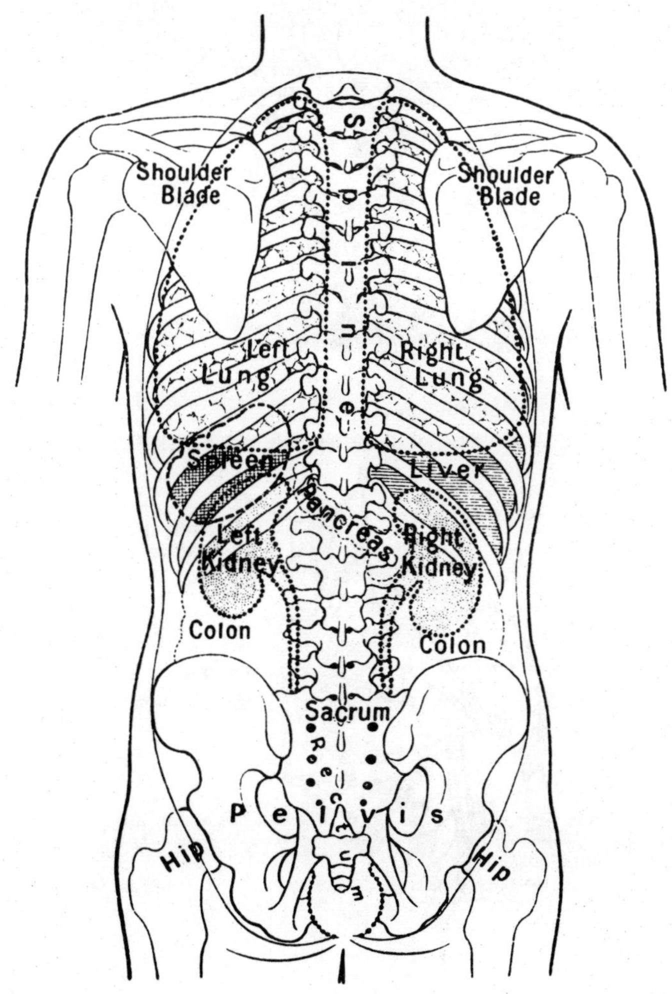

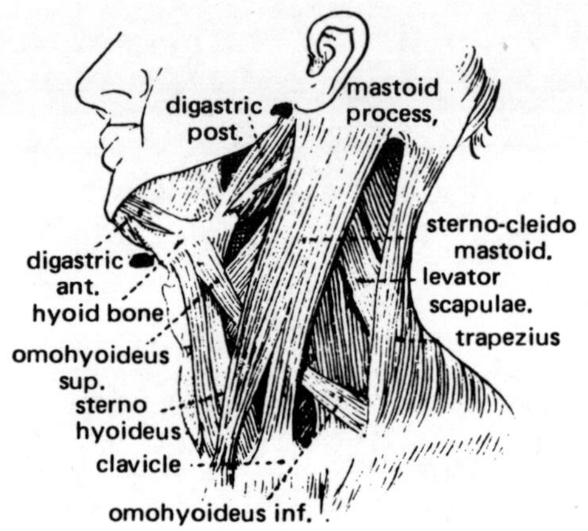

The muscles of the left side of the neck

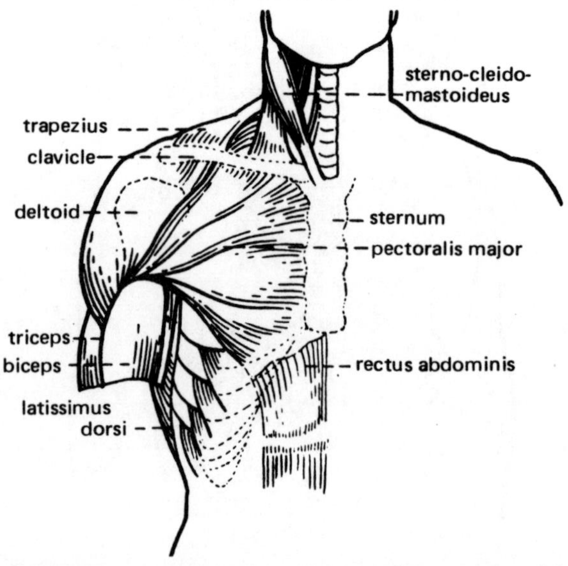

The muscles of the anterior aspect of the shoulder and chest (right)

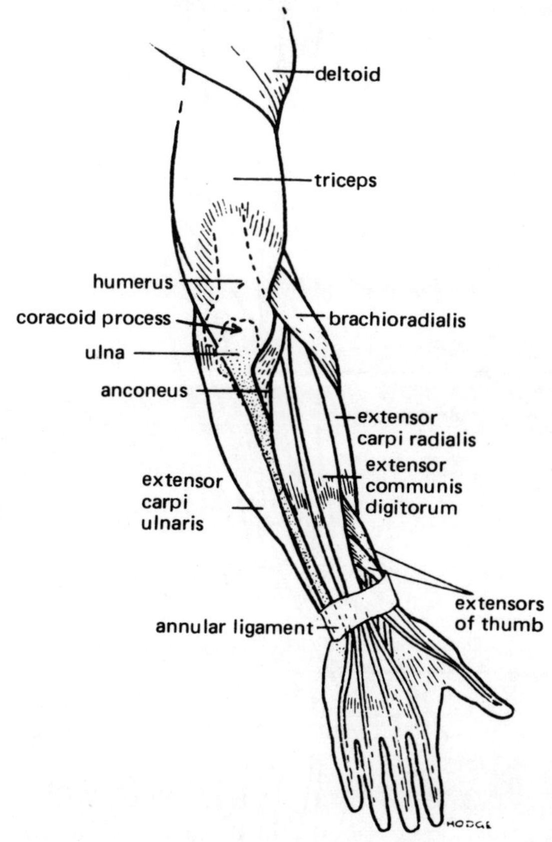

The muscles on the posterior aspect of the forearm (right)

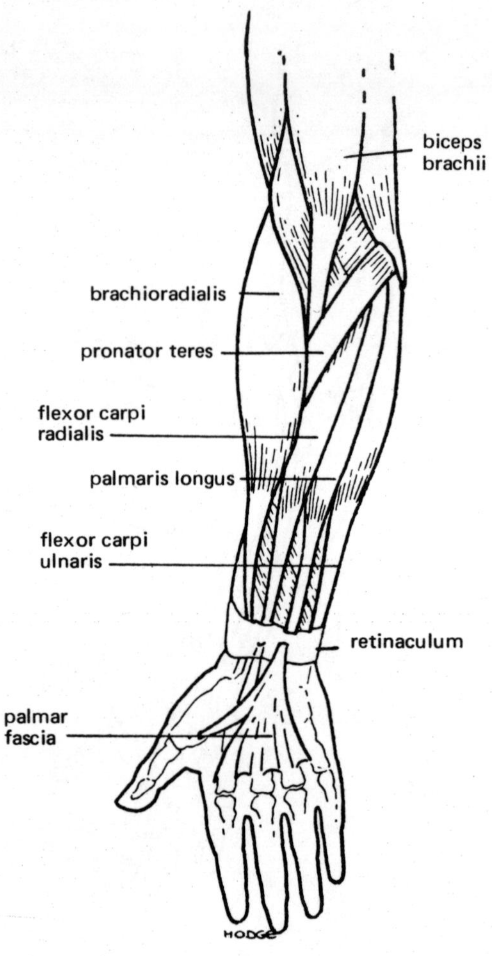

Illustration showing the muscles on the anterior aspect of the forearm (right)

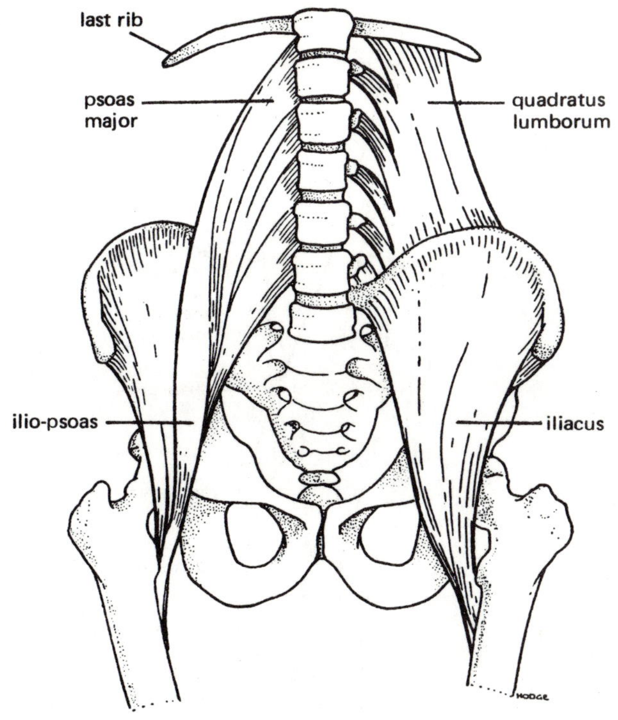

Illustration showing the position of the psoas and iliacus muscles. On the right the blending of the two muscles is shown as they pass to their common insertion on the small trochanter of the femur.

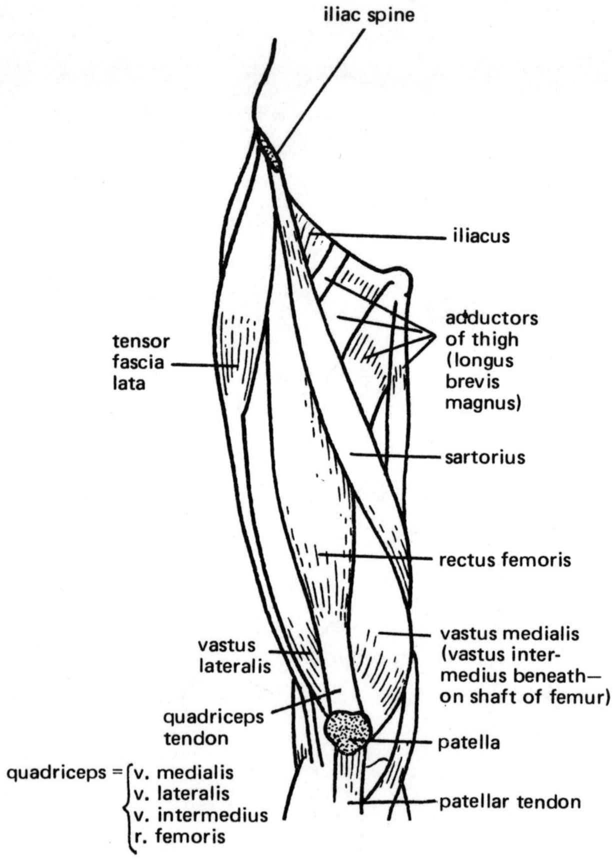

Illustration showing the muscles of the anterior aspect of the thigh (right).

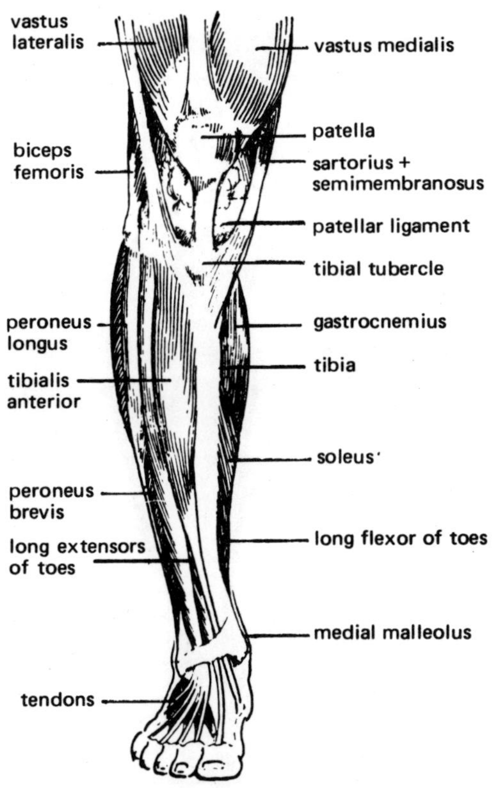

Illustration showing muscles of the leg (anterior)

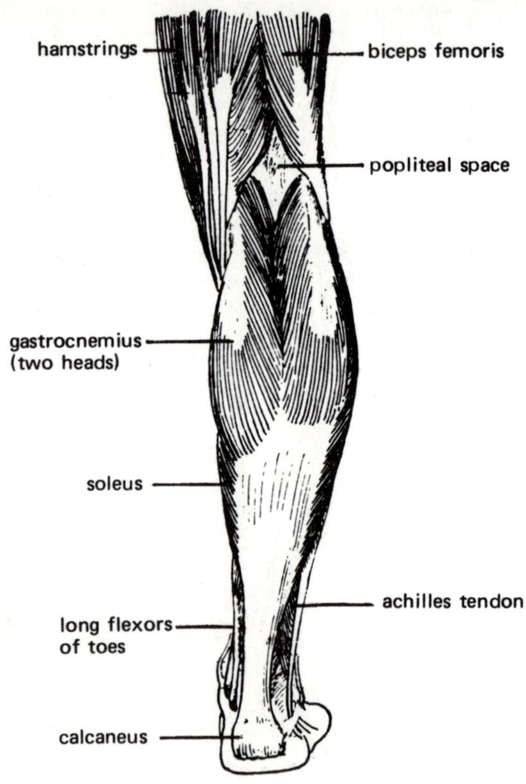

Illustration showing muscle of the leg (posterior)

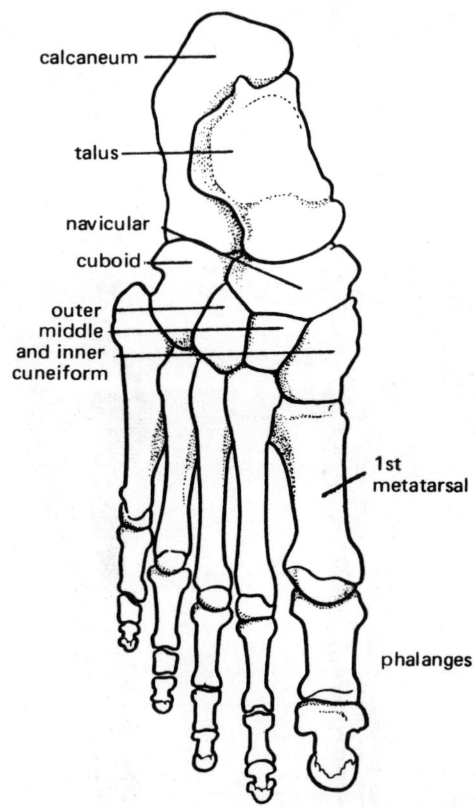

Illustration showing the dorsal aspect of the bones of the right foot.

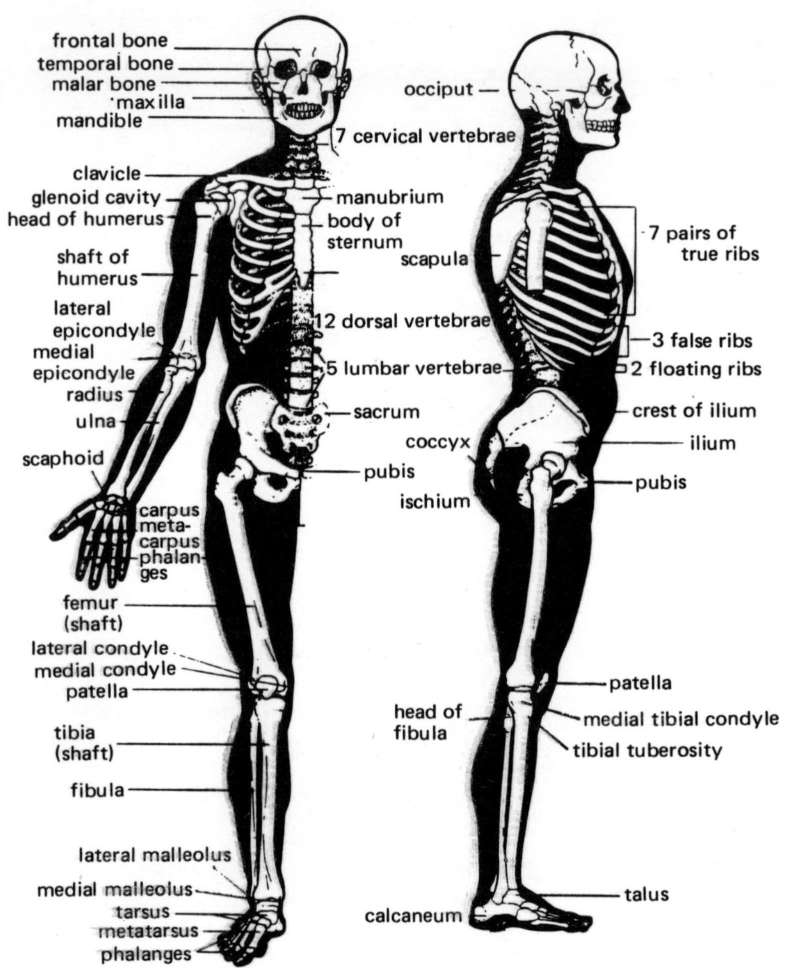

frontal bone
temporal bone
malar bone
maxilla
mandible
7 cervical vertebrae
clavicle
glenoid cavity
head of humerus
manubrium
body of sternum
shaft of humerus
lateral epicondyle
medial epicondyle
radius
ulna
scaphoid
12 dorsal vertebrae
5 lumbar vertebrae
sacrum
pubis
carpus
meta-carpus
phalan-ges
femur (shaft)
lateral condyle
medial condyle
patella
tibia (shaft)
fibula
lateral malleolus
medial malleolus
tarsus
metatarsus
phalanges
occiput
scapula
7 pairs of true ribs
3 false ribs
2 floating ribs
crest of ilium
coccyx
ilium
pubis
ischium
patella
head of fibula
medial tibial condyle
tibial tuberosity
talus
calcaneum

4. FUNCTIONS OF THE BODY
(Physiology)

EXERCISE. An understanding of the changes that occur during exercise in the organs of the body is essential to all coaches, trainers and sports masters.

Exercise is a complex interaction of cardiovascular (heart and vessels), respiratory (lungs), and nervous tissues.

Muscle fibres can only contract in the presence of energy supplied by glucose, which is stored in the muscle as glycogen or transported from the liver by the blood.

Glucose is burnt in oxygen (aerobic metabolism) which diffuses into the tissues from the haemaglobin of the red blood corpuscles. The glucose is converted into carbon dioxide and water. The former is expired by the lungs.

When oxygen is not immediately available glucose is altered to lactic acid (anaerobic metabolism), and the body builds up an oxygen debt. At the end of such an exercise the athlete inhales vast quantities of air to combat this debt and convert the lactic acid to carbon dioxide and water. The 100m and long jump are anaerobic events, no breath is taken during either. In the 200m and 400m races the greatest proportion of energy is obtained from anaerobic metabolism. Thus at high altitudes, where the air is 'thinner' and contains a lower partial pressure of oxygen, the anaerobic races do not suffer and are in fact enhanced by the decreased friction imparted to the moving body (long distant shooting at football becomes more effective, sprinting more rapid). The records produced in the above events at the Mexico Olympics bear testimony to this fact.

To supply the necessary oxygen a great increase in muscle blood flow is needed.

At rest the muscle blood flow is 2ml per 100 grm per minute, during exercise this goes up to 30ml (a fifteen fold increase). The cardiac output per minute rises from 5 litres to 12–20 litres. To produce such an increase the pulse rate would have to rise to 250 plus. This is not practicable because above 180 the heart fills incompletely; it is beating too fast. Therefore some other mechanism is responsible.

Each heart beat ejects 70 mls of blood (the stroke volume), but between 20 and 50 ml remain behind in the ventricles as pooled blood.

With exercise the cardiac muscle develops in size (like ordinary muscle) and the volume of residual blood increases. During activity the heart calls on this pooled blood and the stroke volume goes up to 100–120 ml.

Changes also occur in the respiratory system.

At rest the normal person breathes about 12 times per minute on average and uses 500ml of air per breath (or 6L per minute). During activity this volume goes up to 120L per minute, an increase of 20x. The maximum breathing capacity of an individual is almost double this figure (200L per min), and thus the body has adequate respiratory reserves even during the most severe exercise.

The air, containing 20% oxygen, swirls down the main air-passages (larynx, trachea and bronchi) to the minute, thin-walled air sacs or alveoli. There are 300,000,000 in both lungs, constituting a surface area for absorption of oxygen and liberation of carbon dioxide of 70 square metres (that is 40x the surface area of the body). The oxygen rapidly diffuses into the blood stream and attaches itself to the haemoglobin of the red blood corpuscle (5 million per cc of blood) and is transported to the tissues. The high level of carbon dioxide and other metabolic products produced in the muscles with exercise cause the oxygen to dissociate itself from the red cells and the carbon dioxide is then taken up and carried back to the lungs.

The stimulus to breathing is not primarily oxygen lack but the excess of carbon dioxide and other chemicals (like lactic acid) that alter the acidity (pH) of the blood circulating through the brain. In the medulla oblongata (an area at the base of the brain) the respiratory centre, that controls the rate and depth of respiration, is found. Alterations in carbon dioxide level and pH affect the nerve cells and the respiration is adjusted accordingly.

Respiratory distress occurs as the carbon dioxide accumulates in the blood and alveoli, and second wind follows when this excess is exhaled or when the respiratory centre becomes adjusted to a higher level.

The capacity to transport oxygen by the blood puts a limit to the ability of the sportsman to do work; the limit is placed by the circulation and not by the ability of the lungs to exchange gases. Some experiments suggest that in the muscles there are nerve endings which, on stimulation by metabolites, produce reflexly an increase in respiration. Others maintain that the respiratory centre becomes more sensitive to the above mentioned substances.

The body temperature rises by up to 2F during exercise, and many of the beneficial effects of the warming-up period are said to stem from this increase (as a car functions more smoothly when warm). However a short rest period rapidly dissipates this heat. During activity the heat is lost by sweating and 1L of sweat can be lost in a routine soccer match.

Psychology of an Athlete

Under normal circumstances before an athletic event takes place the brain sends a series of nervous impulses to the adrenal glands, situated one on either side of the abdomen above the kidneys, and the hormones adrenaline and noradrenaline are secreted into the blood stream. These are the hormones of the 'fight or flight' reaction. They promote a discharge of glucose from the liver, an increased mobilisation and utilisation of glucose in the muscles, an increase in pulse and respiratory rate, a slowing down of activity in the bowel and bladder, a shunting of blood from the skin (producing pallor), a facilitation of sweating, a dilatation of the pupils, an increase in the blood supply to the muscles, a heightening of nervous reflexes, and an increased arousal of the individual. ALL these effects are beneficial to the player and improve performance. If excessive, however, the athlete may become paralysed with fear, rapidly using up his glucose stores, and altering the nervous reflexes to produce inco-ordinated muscle actions and hence loss of skill.

Apprehension for weeks or days before the event will also have the same basic effects on the body, and the increased arousal-activity of the brain causes sleepless nights, and a vicious circle ensues. This pre-match apprehension varies from individual to individual—some sportsmen never seem to worry but a rapid pulse and dilated pupil may be give away signs—and the coach must dissipate such stressful circumstances as quickly as possible. Sleep is essential, an evening walk, a warm beverage, a glass of beer, plus a dark, quiet room are most beneficial. In refractory cases sleeping tablets can be used, Mandrax is one of the best since it does not produce a hangover. Often the allocation of bedrooms between a senior, calm player and the nervous junior has a relaxing effect on the latter.

Anxiety may be personal, domestic, social, or have a physical basis. Since athletes rely upon 100% efficiency in performance fears of injury, especially recurrent injury, are always uppermost in their minds. The prompt diagnosis and treatment of such conditions, not only stops simple injuries from becoming chronic insoluble ones, but allays worries and produces confidence in the doctor, coach, or trainer. An optimistic attitude towards the match or event by all concerned is a great incentive to peak performance. This is why a good team spirit is vital for successful results, and an always-cheerful, optimistic player is an asset to any team and worth his place in the party for this reason alone.

The trainer or coach must assess the personality of a player, help to iron out any anxieties and adapt his ability to the needs of the side. Should any problems crop up then a sympathetic discussion and reassurance, combined with a deep interest in these problems, are the greatest aids to overcoming the difficulties. Sedatives, tranquillisers and antidepressants are rarely needed by a sportsman.

Sexual worries are most common in the female, primarily concerned with pregnancy and menstruation. The combined oestrogen/progesterone tablets (the pill) will allay these anxieties, but must be medically prescribed.

Before a match many players follow a strict ritual in the hotel and dressing-room as an omen of good luck, and this ritual should not be interfered with or subjected to ridicule. Similarly the pre-match warm up is beneficial in allowing the players to get the feel of the turf, ball, arena etc. Crepes, dressings and bandages (commonly applied to the knee or wrist) rarely give anatomical support but are good psychologically.

During a match the psychology of gamesmanship comes into play. This is a broad subject and difficult to comment upon. Generally speaking gamesmanship is unethical when it becomes bad manners or ungentlemanly. However there is nothing more demoralising to an exhausted athlete than to see a close competitor cheerfully trotting along, seemingly with pounds of energy to spare. A good example is that of Zatopek, having already won two gold medals in the Olympics, asking the leader of the Marathon, in this case Peters, only a few miles from home, if they were really running fast enough. It is during such exhausting periods that the mustering of the last ounce of effort wins the prize; as Bannister said during his four-minute mile, his mind took control over his body. It is the exceptional athlete who can rise above the stress of fatigue to win an event, the truly professional sportsman.

Finally all coaches should coax rather than bully. Bullying is only successful when accompanied by success. If failures follow then the player becomes resentful of such behaviour.

REMEMBER—A happy athlete is a good athlete.

The Meaning of Fitness

No player or athlete should indulge in maximum activity until fully fit. If, after a long lay-off through injury, exercise produces a recurrence of the injury then all confidence is lost. When undertrained the athlete risks sprained ligaments, pulled muscles from poor co-ordination, and perhaps other injuries from bodily contact with opposing players since fatigue reduces mobility and agility. Overtraining however can lead to chronic damage to tendons (peritendinitis, or recurrent partial tears), ligamentous strains (especially at the ankle or foot), and stress fractures in a variety of bones. Thus fitness is a happy medium between under and overtraining.

But fitness varies according to the sport. 'Fitness for what?' one might ask. Fitness for a sedentary occupation requires only 60% efficiency in locomotor performance, whereas a highly trained athlete needs 100%. A wrestler requires a different degree of fitness to a tennis player, a golfer to a long distance runner. Each sporting activity makes general demands on the heart, lungs, blood vessels, muscles, joints etc., but every sport also makes specific demands on certain organs or structures e.g. the enormous increase in forearm girth of a tennis player or archer, the powerful quadriceps of a footballer or hurdler. The old saying that athletes are born not made has a general ring of truth in it. An analysis of athletes in the last Olympic Games indicated that the greatest percentage belonged to the broad, muscular mesomorphic group, with a small percentage of thin (ectomorphs) in the distance events, and a few fat (endomorphs) in the weights, throwing and similar events. Thus a person's build determines his sporting aptitude. However, once a sport has been adopted then performance depends not only on anatomical and physiological parameters, but includes the degree of training and a will to win. Some players lack the necessary drive and ambition to be successful, either on the field of play, or as self-discipline during training.

Training aims at building up the cardio-vascular and respiratory reserves by a combination of short sprints admixed with longer running, jogging and walking; with an increase in the more severe exercises as the standard of fitness improves. Weight training can then be utilised to increase the muscle mass, i.e. the 'red' fibres, connective and vascular tissues, and at the same time it takes the joints through a full range of movement thus improving the extensibility of tendons and ligaments necessary for peak performance. Straining under heavy weights is useless. Sooner or later chronic strains or multiple small tears will appear to cause disability. Select the maximum comfortable lift for each area concerned and reduce it by 20 lbs. Do NOT carry out a manoeuvre with the weights until a dull pain or aching is produced, this pain indicates minor damage to the structures concerned. After a spell with the weights activity can be resumed, with sprinting to build up the fast-contracting 'white' fibres.

The key to successful training is variety. Some activities are mundane, like lapping around a pitch. A trip on a country run adds interest and a change in surroundings. Some coaches persevere with the same old routine that the players become automated puppets, bored and hardly aware of what is going on. Competitions, by splitting up teams into small groups heightens enjoyment of such activities. Ball games are always fun, and although amongst ball-players stress should always be laid on his/her particular sport, other ball games will give added diversion and training at the same time.

Finally, after injury, all ranges of movement, active and passive, should be tested. Stress can be applied to the upper limb by press-ups and hand-stands, to the back by toe-touching and forming a letter-C with the head towards the heels, and to the lower limbs by hopping on one leg and crouch-springing from the heels in a waddling gait. The pulse and breathing rate can be ascertained after one minute of stepping on and off a 1–2′ stool or box as a means of estimating cardio-respiratory efficiency. There are a lot of other simple tests and providing the coach and trainer becomes familiar with a few and uses them in a standard fashion with each player he can soon assess a return to peak fitness. But the golden rule remains —NEVER rush a player or athlete back to full activity, a gradual increase in performance should be accepted.

5. GENERAL DATA

HEAT...is best given by short wave diathermy, although infra-red and hot baths are used in clubs and schools lacking resources, with good results. Recent injuries must never be heated. Wait at least 48 hours.

PHYSIOTHERAPY...requires skill and does not mean bending and wobbling the parts hopefully. Most trainers, coaches, etc. can attend courses or seek advice from trained physiotherapists.

MASSAGE...is fast becoming obsolete, especially to recent injuries, when more damage is often imparted to the wounded area than was there originally. It is helpful in stiffness, pre-match warm up, and in chronic lesions as deep frictions.

STEROID INJECTIONS...are of use in certain chronic conditions, but must be given accurately. Must never be given into joints (in a fit person) or when tendon tears are detected. They are *not* the panacea for all athletic conditions.

ANALGESICS...despite its ubiquity aspirin still remains one of the most efficient painkillers and anti-inflammatory agents; two tablets, four times a day. Recent drugs, like indomethacin, or phenylbutazone can be used. Oral dispersing agents are used with hope by many large clubs, I remain unconvinced.

ULTRASOUND...is in vogue. Useful in chronic conditions especially pertendinitis and for localising ligamentous tears.

CREPE SUPPORTS have always been in vogue, especially around the knee, where they offer a little support and a great deal of consolation. Have been worn on the normal leg to fool opposition on occasions. If bandaging interferes with the joint action, i.e. limits it, then it is doing some good, if full mobility is allowed then ligaments, tendons etc. can go on being damaged.

WARMING UP requires gently stretching all the key muscle groups in the body by toe touching etc. and not galloping round the pitch which may only affect a few. A car may not function best when cold but the human body is more fortunate, we are always ticking over. Warming up is useful in allaying anxiety. WARMING DOWN is very important, this gentle jogging and walking after an event for 4–5 minutes promotes tissue fluid absorption and helps to prevent stiffness. Elevation of the limbs at half time above waist level will promote a return of fluid from the legs and is beneficial in combatting stiffness and cramps.

DRUGS before an event never win anything but universal condemnation. If a player is not fit a few hours before a match then he never will be, conditions do not clear up in the half-hour before an event. They are usually ignored in the hope of playing and turn simple problems into chronic, insoluble ones.

A GOOD CLUB CARES FOR ITS ATHLETE'S HEALTH AND HAS.....

A stretcher, splints, wooden board or support for spinal injuries,

A supply of varying size crepe and cotton bandages, including triangular bandage.

Sterile dressings of various sizes, cotton-wool, tulle gras, elastoplast and other adhesive plasters.

Adhesive felt-padding.

Mild antiseptic solutions, like dettol, T.C.P., Hibitane etc.

A supply of warm water, and cold ice-cubes (plus towel and polythene bag).

Adrenaline solution for nose bleeds.

Eye bath.

Dumb-bell sutures.

(Black silk sutures, catgut, needles, forceps, scissors etc. for medical attendant).

Aspirins, other analgesics. Antacids for gastric upsets. Anti-diarrhoeal pills for overseas travelling. Occasionally sleeping pills.

Local anaesthetic spray (and in ampoules for doctor).

Syringes and needles (doctor).

Steroids for injection (doctor).

Antibiotic skin sprays, local 'plastic' covering sprays (for abrasions).
Anti-inflammatory tablets (phenylbutazone, indomethacin).
Oral dispersing agents ('Ananase', 'Chymoral' etc.).
Smelling salts, sponge etc. (Trainer's Bag).
and a copy of SPORTS INJURIES, an illustrated manual for trainers, coaches, players, and schools.

DOPING IS:—

1. The administration to or use by a *healthy* individual while taking part in a sporting competition of:—

(a) Any chemical agent or substance not normally present in the body and which does not play either an essential or normal part in the day to day biochemical environment or processes of metabolism, regardless of dosage, preparation or route of administration,

and/or

(b) Any chemical agent or substance which plays an essential or normal part in the day to day processes of metabolism or forms a normal part of the biochemical environment, when introduced in abnormal quantities and/or by an abnormal route and/or in abnormal form,

either or both of which (a. and/or b.) are present in the body of the individual during competition for the PURPOSE or with the EFFECT of modifying artificially the performance of the individual during competition.

DOPING IS ALSO:—

2. The administration to or use by an individual temporarily or permanently *disabled* by disease or injury who takes part in a sporting competition of:—

(c) Any chemical agent or substance regardless of nature, dosage, preparation or route of administration, for the sole purpose of alleviating or curing the disability and/or its cause,

which, being present in the body of the individual during competition would, BY ITS SECONDARY effects improve artificially the performance of that individual during competition.

The following drug substances must never be used for the *treatment* of sportsmen and sportswomen while they are actually taking part in sports competitions.

Alcohol (specifically ethyl alcohol):

Amphetamines and their derivatives.

Purine bases.

Camphor and pharmaco-dynamically similar substances, including the Analeptics.

Cocaine.

Digitalin and similar substances.

Monoamine oxidase inhibitors.

Lobelline and similar substances.

Nitrites and similar substances—peripheral vasodilators.

Phenothiazines.

Picrotoxine.

Narcotics.

Strychnine.

Tropeines.

Uridine triphosphate.

Hormones (including those of the corticosteroid and allied series).

Hormones (including those of the corticosteroid and allied series) when given systematically, unless they have been *regularly* used by the patient for the previous 28 days or longer.*

* The use of steroids for suppression of the menstrual period in female competitors may be taken to be excluded from this ban pending further clarification and international discussion.

B.A.S.M. POLICY STATEMENT ON DOPING PUBLISHED 1964 *

Bearing in mind the many implications of the use of chemical agents of one kind or another to modify artificially the performance of healthy human beings not only in sport but in all walks of life, the British Association of Sport and Medicine considers and recommends that:—

1. The only effective and safe way of ensuring optimum performance in any activity is a proper programme of training and preparation.
2. No known chemical agent is capable of producing both safely and effectively an improvement in performance in a healthy human subject.
3. Every chemical agent taken by the healthy human subject with the intention of artificially improving his performance is in some degree harmful to the individual who takes it.
4. No purpose (other than medical—therapeutic or prophylactic) is properly to be served by the administration or use of chemical agents with the intention or effect of modifying human performance, except in cases of properly controlled experiment and research.
5. The use of chemical agents other than for medical purposes shall be regarded as DOPING. A full definition of DOPING is set out in the first appendix to this draft.
6. DOPING should be actively discouraged, and Governing Bodies of Sport and other interested parties should consider and implement what steps they can take appropriate to this end.
7. The public advertisement of chemical agents or preparations for purposes which fall within the definition of DOPING should cease and Parliamentary legislation to this end should be sought if necessary.
8. Appropriate methods should be evolved actively to curb the practise of DOPING, such methods to include an educational campaign, the prohibition of DOPING in the

rules of Sports generally, the application of sanctions to offenders, and the introduction of suitable methods of test and control.

9. When a sportsman or woman is taking part in a competition while receiving drugs of any kind as a form of properly authorised medical treatment, the same should be made known in confidence to the duly authorised representatives of the body organising the competition.

10. No drug included in the list shown in the second appendix to this draft shall ever be used for the properly authorised medical treatment of any individual taking part in a sporting competition and where the use of any such prohibited drug is medically necessary the sportsman or woman concerned must be withdrawn from that competition.

The British Association of Sport and Medicine further considers that should its recommendations be put into effect the results can only be to the benefit of sport in particular, and the health of the community in general.

* Published by permission of The British Association of Sports and Medicine.

INDEX

Abdomen, injuries, 62
Achilles tendon rupture, 88-90
peritendinitis, 92
Acromioclavicular joint injuries, 38, 40, 41
Anatomy, 112-24
Ankle, injuries, 93-5
Anterior tibial compartment syndrome, 90
Arm, injuries, 45-8
Arterial damage, diagnosis, 11
Artificial respiration, 4-5

Baker's cyst, 85
Baseball elbow, 52
Bennett fracture, 56, 58
Biceps rupture (arm), 45
Blisters, 97
Bone (structure), 110, 111
Brachial neuralgia, 45
Brain injury, 27-9

Calcaneum, fractures, 97
Cartilages (damage), knee, 80
structure, 101
cyst, 81
Chest, injuries, 60-61
Chondromalacia patellae, 72, 74
Clavicle, injuries, 37-40
Colles fracture, 53, 54
Connective tissue, 99

Damage—see under structure (e.g. muscle, knee, etc.)
Dislocation—see under structure (e.g. mandible, elbow)
diagnosis, 8
Doping, BASM policy statement, 138

Elbow, injuries, 49
dislocation, 49
Emergency treatment, 1-5
Exercise, function, 125
External cardiac massage, 5
Extradural haemorrhage, 27

Facial injuries, 31
Femur, fractures, 65-6
Fibula, fractures, 90
Finger, injuries, 56-9
Fitness, 131
Footballer's ankle, 95
Foot injuries, 96, 97-8
Fracture—see under structure (e.g. skull, arm, etc.)
diagnosis, 6
Frozen shoulder, 41

General data, 134
Golfer's elbow, 52

Hallux valgus, 97
Head injuries, 23
Hip injuries, 64-5
Humerus, fractures, 45-8

Ingrowing toe nail, 97
Injury—see under structure (e.g. skin, bone, etc.)
Intermuscular injury, 18
Intramuscular injury, 18

Javelin elbow, 52
Joints—see under structure (e.g. elbow, knee), 101-103
function and recording, 103

Kidney injury, 62
Knee, dislocation, 72
injuries, 70-89

Leg injuries, 90-92
Ligament injury, 15
knee, 70-89
Ligaments, ankle, 93
Liver injuries, 62

Malar fracture, 31
Mallet finger, 57
Mandible, fracture, 31
dislocation, 32
Medial ligament damage (knee), 75-7, 79, 81-2
Meniscal damage (knee), 80
Muscle, damage, 18-22
structure, 109, 111
Muscles of the body, 116-22
Myositis ossificans, 21, 22, 48

Nerve damage, diagnosis, 13

Olecranon, fracture, 49
Osgood-Schlatter's disease, 85
Osteoarthritis, knee, 85
Osteochondritis dissecans (elbow), 52
(knee), 73, 74

Patellar bursae, 85
Patella, injuries, 72-3
Pelvis, injuries, 64
Peritendinitis, 17
Plantaris, rupture, 90
Plantar fasciitis, 97
Potts fracture, 93-4
Prolapse of intervertebral disc, 36, 45
Psychology of an athlete, 128
Pulled hamstrings, 68
Pulled gastrocnemius, 90

Radius (head) fracture, 49
(shaft) fracture, 53
Recurrent groin injury, 66-7
Ribs, fracture, 60

Scaphoid, fracture, 56
Scapula, fracture, 37, 38
Semimembranosus bursa, 85
Shoulder, dislocation, 41, 42
injury, 41-3
Skeleton (bone structure), 124
Skin, injury, 14-15
structure, 99-100
Skull fracture, 23-9
Spinal injuries, 33-6
Spleen, injury, 62
Subdural harmorrhage, 28
Supracondylar fracture, 47-8
Supraspinatus tears, 41-3

Tendon injury, 16-17
Tennis elbow, 49-50
Tenosynovitis, 17
wrist, 55
ankle, 93
Testicular injury, 62
Thigh injuries, 66-8
Tibial fractures, 90-91

Unconscious player, emergency care, 3
Urethra, injury, 62